W9-BTQ-262

Photo/Illustration credits:

Figure 1.1 *Courtesy of Westwood Pharmaceuticals Inc.*

Figure 1.2 Upper Left: Courtesy of Jack Weisbach; Upper Right: Courtesy of Eastman Kodak Company. Reproduced from "Skin Cancer: Preventable and Curable," a slide presentation. ©1988 The Skin Cancer Foundation.

Figure 2.1 Reproduced from "Skin Cancer: Preventable and Curable," a slide presentation. ©1988, The Skin Cancer Foundation.

Figure 4.1 Reproduced from "Skin Cancer: Preventable and Curable," a slide presentation. ©1988, The Skin Cancer Foundation.

Figure 4.2 Reproduced from "Skin Cancer: Preventable and Curable," a slide presentation. ©1988, The Skin Cancer Foundation.

Figure 5.1 Courtesy of Eclipse Laboratories.

Figure 6.1 Courtesy of Westwood Pharmaceuticals Inc.

Figure 7.1 Courtesy of the Food and Drug Administration, U.S. Department of Health and Human Services.

Figure 8.1 Reprinted with permission of The American Pharmaceutical Association. ©1988 Mark Farris.

Figure 8.2 Courtesy of Eastman Kodak Company.

Figure 8.3 Reproduced from "Skin Cancer: Preventable and Curable," a slide presentation. ©1988, The Skin Cancer Foundation.

Figures 16.1 through 16.6 Illustrations by Monika Bittman.

Illustrations by Howard Roberts: 3.1, 9.1, 13.1, chart page 194, and 21.1.

Color section:

Photos 1 – 6 Reproduced from "Basal Cell Carcinoma: The Most Common Cancer," ©1986, The Skin Cancer Foundation.

Photos 7 – 11 Reproduced from "Squamous Cell Carcinoma: The Second Most Common Skin Cancer," ©1990, The Skin Cancer Foundation.

Photo 12 Reproduced from "Skin Cancer: Preventable and Curable," a slide presentation. ©1988, The Skin Cancer Foundation.

Photo 13 Reproduced from "The ABCD's of Moles and Melanomas," ©1985, The Skin Cancer Foundation.

Photo 14 Reproduced from "The Many Faces of Malignant Melanoma," ©1985, 1987, The Skin Cancer Foundation.

Photo 15 Reproduced from "Skin Cancer: Preventable and Curable," a slide presentation. ©1988, The Skin Cancer Foundation.

Photo 16 Reproduced from "Skin Cancer: Preventable and Curable," a slide presentation. ©1988, The Skin Cancer Foundation.

FOREWORD

Dr. Perry Robins is President of The Skin Cancer Foundation and an experienced dermatologic surgeon who has pioneered the Mohs micrographic surgical technique for the treatment of cancers of the skin. In this book he explains in layman's terms the devastating effects that radiation from the sun can produce in the skin.

While the emphasis of this book is on precancers and cancers of the skin, it also delves into other important consequences of too much exposure to the sun, namely, photosensitive skin diseases and "photoaging." Photoaging is a combination of blotchy discolorations of the skin, wrinkling, and sagging tissues, all of which combine to produce prematurely "aged" skin.

The fundamental message from Dr. Robins is that the down side of exposure to solar radiation can be prevented by adopting rather simple protective measures, such as application of sunscreens and wearing clothing that blocks the sun.

Another important goal of this book is to encourage the reader to begin a program of self-examination of the skin. In easily understood diagrams, this process is clearly identified. Detection of early cancers of the skin allows prompt removal and cure. This is especially important for malignant melanoma, which is a potentially fatal type of skin cancer. In contrast, delayed diagnosis of melanoma (for whatever reasons) can allow the cancer to advance to a point where it spreads to other organs of the body (metastasizes), a process that often leads to very serious consequences.

The generous use of charts, diagrams, and photographs included here aids the reader in identifying precancerous and cancerous lesions of the skin.

This book is for you! Complicated medical terminology is largely avoided, and simple, practical suggestions are made for sun protection appropriate for all age groups. You will learn how to avoid the ravaging rays of the sun and to identify those conditions and diseases that are caused by sunlight so that they can be properly diagnosed and treated.

The book ends on a note of promise of things to come in the future based on current and future research. Understanding the biologic changes that occur as a consequence of solar radiation will mean better approaches to diagnosis and treatment. The research of today is the promise for a better future.

Finally, Dr. Robins, in his unique experience as a practitioner of dermatologic surgery, educator at all

Sun Sense

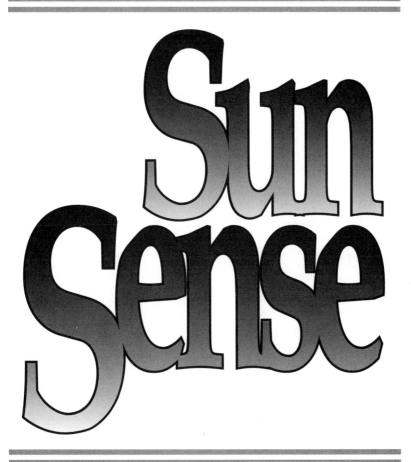

Sun Sense

Perry Robins, M.D.

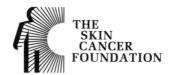

THE
SKIN
CANCER
FOUNDATION

The goal of this book is to provide accurate and practical medical information to the general reader. However, its contents are not intended to offer medical advice on individual health problems, which should be obtained directly from a physician. We regret that we cannot respond to inquiries regarding personal health matters.

Book Design by H. Roberts

ISBN 0-9627688-0-4

Printed in the United States of America

levels, administrator, and philanthropist, has demonstrated once again his total dedication to improving skin health and preventing or properly treating precancers and cancers of the skin. We all owe a debt of gratitude to Dr. Robins for his continuing and untiring efforts to help us enjoy better skin health.

Alfred W. Kopf, M.D.
Clinical Professor
Department of Dermatology
New York University
School of Medicine

ACKNOWLEDGMENTS

First and foremost, I would like to express my appreciation to my collaborator, Linda Tarlton, a gifted writer and researcher, who spent countless hours and many months working with me on this manuscript. Her contribution is immense. I also want to thank the many fellows who have worked with me in the past and who have contributed to this book: namely, Calvin L. Day, Jr., M.D., Roy Geronemus, M.D., Deborah Sarnoff, M.D., David J. Goldberg, M.D., Carl Vinciullo, M.D., Blas A. Reyes, M.D., Isaack Zilinsky, M.D., Richard G. Bennett, M.D., and Mark Hassell, M.D. I am also indebted to my colleague René Rodriguez-Sains, M.D., for his input in ophthalmology, to Drs. Jean-Claude Bystryn, Darrell S. Rigel, and Jason Rivers for their expertise on melanoma, and to Dr. Madhukar A. Pathak, for his contributions in the area of photobiology. Dr. Alfred W. Kopf, whose guidance and counsel have been invaluable to me through the years, has been of immeasurable help in reviewing and editing portions of the book.

The public information staff of The Skin Cancer Foundation (Joyce Weisbach Ayoub, Teri Barr, Barbara Ravage, and Barbara Black) are to be commended for their support and ongoing commitment to the education of millions of people on the subject of skin cancer. I want especially to acknowledge Mitzi Moulds, Executive Director, The Skin Cancer Foundation, whose inspired leadership and dedication has made the vision of this Foundation a reality.

I am grateful to the staff of the Journal Publishing Group, Roberta Fineman (Publications Director), Beverly Byrne, Jennifer Koch-Weser, and Elizabeth Mozden for unselfishly volunteering their time and considerable talent to the production and publication of this manuscript; Howard Roberts for his excellent art direction; and Dorothy Segal and Mark Yaslow for their editorial input.

Working with me, and the many people involved in the development and publication of this book, is Anne Akers, who has made this book happen and to whom I express sincere appreciation.

My office and nursing staff, Maryann Azzaritti, Sheri Frank, Stacey Gelband, Donna Gravina, Lisa Marie Jimenez, Mariae Lane, Harriet Schachtman, Marie Tudisco, and Susan Young, also deserve particular mention. For many years they have rendered tender and concerned care to each and every one of our patients, and even sometimes to me. I appreciate you.

And lastly, my deepest gratitude to my very good friends, Mr. and Mrs. Thomas Langbert and Mr. Joseph Gaumont, who have generously provided the funding to make this book possible.

DEDICATION

To my patients, and to my much beloved children, Elizabeth and Larry Robins.

CONTENTS

CHAPTER 3. THE SUN: CAUSE OF OVER
90% OF SKIN CANCERS
Ultraviolet Radiation / 24
Factors That Influence Solar Radiation / 26
Season / 26
Time of Day / 27
Latitude / 27
Altitude / 27
Climatic and Environmental Conditions / 28

CHAPTER 4. THE OZONE CRISIS / 31

CHAPTER 5. DYING FOR A TAN: NO TAN IS A SAFE TAN
The "Sunshine Vitamin" — How Much Do You Need? / 37
When Sun Strikes Skin: Tanning and Burning / 38
Tanning / 39
Sunburn / 40
Repeated Sun Exposure: The Damage Adds Up / 40
Photosensitivity Reactions / 42

CHAPTER 6. SUN SUSCEPTIBILITY: DETERMINING
YOUR DANGER POINT
What's My Skin Type / 45
Minimal Erythema Dose / 47
Sun Affinity Ratio / 50
Using the Information: Sunscreens and SPF / 50

CHAPTER 7. ARTIFICIAL SUN: SUNLAMPS AND
TANNING BOOTHS
Parlor Operators: "Sunlamps are Safe!" / 55
The Medical Point of View: "Tanning Spells Trouble" / 59
Regulations for Parlors / 60
How to Protect Yourself / 61

CHAPTER 13. WHO GETS SKIN CANCER: THE DIFFERENCES BETWEEN MEN AND WOMEN

CHAPTER 14. SKIN CANCER TREATMENT: WHAT ARE THE OPTIONS?

CHAPTER 15. THE HEALING PROCESS: AFTER SKIN CANCER TREATMENT

INTRODUCTION

A young woman in her mid-thirties recently came to my office concerned about a blemish on her nose. After examining her, I gently explained that the blemish was skin cancer. As I spoke, she sat listening silently, staring into space. Her face grew whiter as I talked. Then her confusion, fear, and anger erupted in a torrent of words:

"What do you mean...skin cancer? You're kidding. You must be wrong. I can't have it."

She paused. "Oh, my God! My friend's mother had it. Do you know what happened to her? It spread, and she ended up dying from it. Will that happen to me? Am I going to lose my nose? Am I going to die?"

She began to cry, and I patted her shoulder, reassuring her that neither was likely. As the anger subsided and the initial impact of what I had told her began to wear off, she regained some of her self-control and began to ask the questions that most of my patients do.

"Why did I get skin cancer? Can it be treated? How?

Will you operate on my nose? What will I look like afterward? Will I be deformed?

When I first began to specialize in cancers of the skin some 25 years ago, there weren't good answers to many of these questions. Today I have answers, not only as they apply to this patient but to other patients with skin cancers as well. During those decades, while I have been at the New York University Medical Center—practicing, teaching, and doing research—new methods of diagnosis and treatment have evolved, along with a better understanding of what causes skin cancer.

Most people don't realize that cancer of the skin is the most common form of cancer. Its incidence is increasing dramatically throughout the world, and it is now developing in younger people. Most of the patients I saw with skin cancer 20 years ago were elderly. Now I find myself operating on malignant lesions in young and middle-aged people. In 1970, the average age of my patients was 65. Today, it is 56.

The major reason that more of us are getting skin cancer, and at an earlier age, has a lot to do with our newly acquired affluence and leisure time—and what we do with it. We spend much of our leisure time in the sun, and with jet travel, we can get to sunny places a lot faster and a lot more often than ever before. The result: more skin cancer.

What cigarettes are to lung cancer, the sun is to skin cancer: the chief cause of this self-induced, largely preventable disease. The dangers are especially high for fair-skinned people, who have a 1 in 3 chance of getting skin cancer. But all of us, whatever our complexion, need to develop more sun sense. Unless we do, skin cancer will take an ever greater toll.

1

SKIN CANCER:
A Vital Concern
for 1 Out of 6
Americans

Cancer—the very word strikes dread into the hearts and minds of most people. Skin cancer, like other kinds of cancer, is a serious disorder. It can cause disfigurement and even death.

But skin cancer differs from many other cancers in several important ways:

- **First, it is visible.** The fact that it is on the skin, not hidden away in internal organs, means it can potentially be detected almost as soon as it begins.
- **Second, it is curable.** Skin cancer has an 85%–99% cure rate.
- **Third, it is preventable.** The vast majority of cases could have been prevented by taking a few simple precautions.

TYPES OF SKIN CANCER

The three most common forms of skin cancer are basal

Types of Skin Cancer

Basal Cell Carcinoma

Squamous Cell Carcinoma

Malignant Melanoma

cell carcinomas, squamous cell carcinomas, and malignant melanomas. Each is named for the type of skin cell from which it originates and has a characteristic appearance and growth pattern.

Basal cell carcinoma is the most common form of skin cancer, accounting for approximately 500,000 new cases annually in the United States. Although basal cell carcinoma rarely metastasizes (spreads to other locations in the body), it is sometimes hard to eradicate, and attempts to completely remove it may mean loss of the nose, eye, or another organ. The tumor generally begins as a small, translucent, pearly bump.

Squamous cell carcinoma is the second most common form of skin cancer; 100,000 cases per year are reported in the United States. Squamous cell carcinomas are pink, tan, or brown, and are opaque, forming either bumps or patches. Although less common than basal cell cancers, they grow faster, and are more likely to spread. Both basal cell and squamous cell carcinomas appear most often on sun-exposed areas of the body.

Malignant melanomas are responsible for most of the deaths due to skin cancer. They may look like moles—small

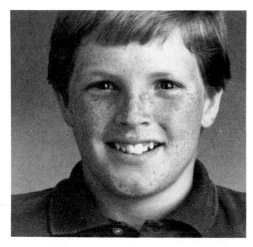

(Figure 1.1)
People who always burn, never tan, and are fair with red or blond hair and freckles have a greater chance of developing skin cancer.

brown-black bumps—or may be larger, multicolored patches; most have irregular borders. Malignant melanoma is a relatively rare but potentially fast-growing form of skin cancer that metastasizes rapidly.

INCIDENCE

In the United States today, there are more than 600,000 new cases of skin cancer diagnosed each year as compared with slightly over one million new cases of all other types of cancer combined. By the year 2010, more than one million cases of skin cancer are expected to occur each year.

One in 6 Americans will eventually develop skin cancer; for those who are fair-haired and light-skinned, the rate increases to 1 in 3 (Figure 1.1). In the years to come, as we begin to see the effects of the dwindling ozone layer, we can predict an even more devastating incidence, occurring at earlier ages. Such a trend is already apparent in my practice.

CAUSES OF SKIN CANCER

Awareness is growing that many cases of skin cancer are brought about by carcinogens—elements in our environment that cause a normal cell to become cancerous. Some chemicals have this potential, as do x-rays, but the most important carcinogen is the sun itself.

Carcinogens are no strangers to the medical profession. In England, as early as 1775, Sir Percival Potts noted a high rate of scrotal cancer in chimney sweeps; he showed that soot was the carcinogenic agent. By the early 1800s coal tar (contained in tobacco-curing agents and snuff) had been incriminated as the cause of lip and mouth cancers.

Radium, once used in fluorescent clock faces and watch dials, induced cancers of the mouth and fingers of workers who dipped their brushes in paint and licked or stroked the brushes to a point before illuminating the numbers.

Chemicals

In the late 1800s, the dermatologist Sir Jonathan Hutchinson first described skin cancers in patients who had been treated with arsenic-containing medicines (a common practice at the time). Although these medicines are no longer in use, dermatologists still sometimes see elderly patients who suffer skin cancer caused by their administration. Gardeners who worked with arsenicals and copper smelters exposed to arsenical fumes suffered similar effects, and inhabitants of geographic areas where well water has a naturally high arsenic content (such as Argentina, Taiwan, and Silesia) also have a high incidence of skin cancer.

With the spread of industry and technology, more and more agents, casually adopted, have proven hazardous and even life-threatening. The list is alarming: many solvents, glues, insulating and packing materials, food preservatives and additives, dyes and coloring agents, herbicides and pesticides, and propellants and cleaning agents. Unfortunately, it often takes years for carcinogenic potential to reveal itself, and new, potentially carcinogenic substances are being introduced every day.

X-Rays

Since 1902, we have known that x-rays can cause cancer. Before this was common knowledge, children's feet were routinely x-rayed by a process called fluoroscopy to determine proper fitting of new shoes. Dental x-rays were also taken routinely with little or inadequate precaution. Dentists, who often casually held the small x-ray film in position in the patient's mouth, suffered the consequences years later: skin cancer of the fingers.

Today, x-rays are taken far less frequently and are of much lower intensity. Lead shields drape the area of the patient's body that needs to be protected. Dentists, radiologists, and assistants trigger the film exposure from outside the room (or from lead-lined booths) to prevent constant exposure to the damaging rays. As few radiographs as possible are taken in children or in women who are pregnant or of childbearing age.

The Sun

It is ironic that the sun, the life-giving force, is also a perilous enemy, the prime cause of most skin cancer. The ultraviolet radiation it emits is a potent carcinogen.

The sun's role in the development of skin cancer cannot be denied. Ninety percent of all skin cancer occurs on sun-exposed parts of the body (Figure 1.2). The face, nose, ears,

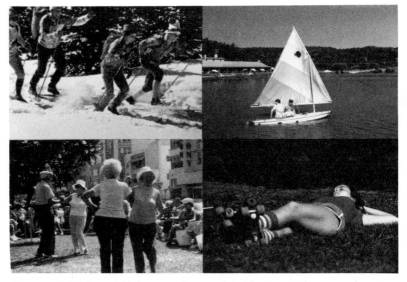

(Figure 1.2) Anyone who spends considerable time in the sun or lives in a sunny climate may develop skin cancer.

neck, and the backs of the hands are particularly vulnerable. Most lip cancers develop on the protruding lower lip, which is less protected from direct sunlight. The eyelids are also especially susceptible. Skin cancer of the nipples, abdomen, buttocks, palms, and soles is much less common.

People who spend a great deal of time outdoors have a greater risk of skin cancer. Fishermen, farmers, ranchers, sailors, construction workers, and athletes all have an incidence of skin cancer greater than that in indoor workers.

Skin cancer is more prevalent in the sunbelt areas of the United States and in tropical and subtropical regions of the world where the sun's rays are more direct, and thus more intense. Perhaps because they are more aware of the dangers of too much sun, people who live in such climates often restrict outdoor activities during the hottest, sunniest hours of the day. They sometimes carry parasols or wear broad-brimmed hats and clothing designed to shield them from the unrelenting sun.

Of increasing concern today is the diminishing ozone layer, the stratospheric shield that protects us from much ultraviolet radiation.

Skin Pigment and Skin Types

Melanin, the naturally occurring pigment present in the uppermost skin layer, is the body's natural defense against the sun's ultraviolet light. Melanin is stimulated by ultraviolet light to rise to the outer layers of the skin, the epidermis, darkening the skin and rendering it somewhat less vulnerable to light absorption. Albinos, who are at very high risk for skin cancer, congenitally lack the capacity to produce melanin and thus have no natural sun shield. Asiatic peoples, Indians, and blacks have greater amounts of melanin in varying degrees and are less susceptible to sun damage, although they can be burned by the sun and do develop skin cancer.

Skin is generally classified into six types, from extremely fair to black. Persons who are light-haired, fair-skinned, and blue-eyed are far more likely to burn and have the greatest risk for skin cancer.

Other Factors

Certain skin conditions and diseases such as porphyria, lupus erythematosus, psoriasis, vitiligo, and photosensitivity may be triggering factors that place individuals at greater risk of developing skin cancer.

Some types of skin cancer seem to run in families, suggesting a genetic component, and the fact that rates are different in men and women point to a hormonal influence. Skin cancer sometimes develops in sites of previous skin damage—ulcers, scar tissue, burns, or tattoos.

TREATMENTS

Striking progress has been made in the area of skin cancer treatment. Today the exact extent of tumor growth can be pinpointed with far greater accuracy than was the case only a few years ago. Progress in plastic and reconstructive surgery now allows correction of defects or scars once considered irreparable.

The most widely used methods today are removal of the tumor by surgery or by radiation therapy. Other methods include removal using an electric needle, chemotherapy, and Mohs micrographic surgery, a microscopically controlled technique that offers unparalleled advantages in certain cases. In the future, lasers, genetic engineering, and immunotherapy may join this arsenal.

PREVENTION

Although we are unable to control many of the causative factors of skin cancer, we can, by simple methods, shield our bodies from one prime factor, the damaging rays of the sun.

Education is the chief means of preventing skin cancer—in essence, reversing the widespread misconceptions that hours in the sunshine are conducive to health and that a golden tan makes a person look not only glamorous but "healthy." Already, education programs are having an effect.

CHAPTER

2

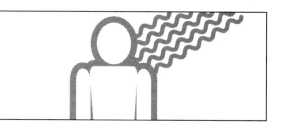

THE SKIN: Our Protective Covering

T

he skin is the body's largest organ, comprising about 10%–15% of adult body weight. If it were laid out, it would extend over almost 20 square feet. It contains myriad nerves; hair follicles; a superabundance of blood vessels; and two or three million sweat glands, which produce both oil (sebum) and sweat.

The skin is more than a passive body covering. It shields internal organs against physical or bacterial injury, actively maintains a constant body temperature, and as a sensory organ alerts us to potential dangers.

THE LAYERS OF THE SKIN

The skin, like other organs, is composed of many different types of cells, each with its own function. Skin cells are arranged in a generally vertical manner, forming a layered structure. Taken together, the outermost layer is the epidermis; the middle layer the dermis; and the deepest layer, the subcutis (fatty layer).

The epidermis seals in body fluids, aids in healing, gives rise to sweat glands and hair follicles, and protects the dermis and internal organs from damage. In the deepest layer of the epidermis are located the basal cells—those that are the foundation, or basic, layer of the skin. Above these are the squamous cells, and finally, in the skin surface, the horny layer. Also found in the epidermis are melanocytes, cells specialized to produce melanin, the principal pigment that colors skin, hair, and eyes.

The epidermis is of major concern to those who are interested in skin cancer because most skin cancers develop from the basal cells, squamous cells, and melanocytes located there (Figure 2.1).

The outer layer of the epidermis, the covering we see, is the stratum corneum, which consists of inert, protein-filled cells called corneocytes. These cells form a tough, waterproof outer coating. The stratum corneum is in a constant state of change. Continuously, dead cells are sloughed off from the top while new cells move up from underneath. We rarely notice this sloughing-off process except on the scalp, the dead cells of which we call dandruff.

Beneath the epidermis is the second layer of the skin, the dermis. The dermis is the support layer of the skin, giving it flexibility and strength. A dense, interwoven network of collagen fibers and elastic, it serves as a support structure for blood and lymph vessels, nerve endings, and muscle fibers. Hair follicles, sweat, and other glands are also rooted there. Fully one-third of all blood circulating in the body is used to nourish the skin, so the blood vessels of the dermis are extremely important to the health of the whole body. Below the dermis is the subcutis, essentially a fat pad that provides insulation, nutrition, and resiliency.

Cross Section of the Skin

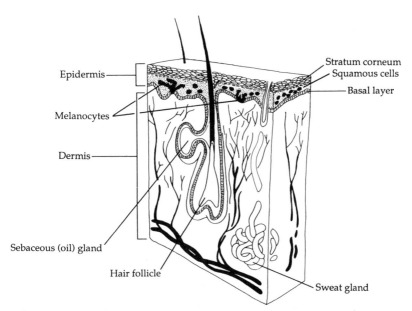

(Figure 2.1) With each exposure to ultraviolet radiation, damage occurs beneath the surface of the skin—damage that does not heal.

The skin varies considerably according to the part of the body where it is located, being very thin on the face and eyelids and thickest on the palms and soles. Nails are an especially thick layer of hard keratin; hair is a threadlike filament of a similar hard keratin.

THE SKIN AS A BARRIER TO INJURY

The skin's construction suits it ideally for its function as a barrier. At an assault such as a scrape, burn, or cut, the skin's blood vessels first tighten up, restricting flow and reducing blood loss. Then they relax. The resulting increase in permeability and fluid seepage in the area around the vessels is a second defense mechanism, the swelling causing a thickening of the stratum corneum to protect against further assault. Sweat glands help clear the body of waste materials and chemical substances.

THE SKIN'S PIGMENTATION

Normal skin comes in a wide range of colors, from the pale skin characteristic of many Northern Europeans to the darkest black. To a large extent, the color of our skin is genetically determined by the amount of melanin our skin produces.

The skin's melanin functions as a shield against the ultraviolet rays of the sun. People with much epidermal melanin are better protected from these rays; those with little are far less so.

THE SKIN AS A REGULATOR OF BODY TEMPERATURE

In addition to its role as a barrier, the skin plays a major role in maintaining body temperature. The human body is designed to function optimally at a constant temperature of 98.6°F. The skin helps maintain this temperature through its sweat glands—small, convoluted tubules that traverse the skin's inner layers, opening to its outer surface.

As the muscles of our bodies work and generate heat, body temperature begins to rise. Vasodilation, an increase in the size of the capillaries and in blood flow through them, conducts heat outward to the skin, where it can be removed from the body. Perspiration also helps cool the body. When we perspire, the water released evaporates into the air, making us feel cooler. This is why we tend to feel cool when we come out of the water after swimming, even when the ambient temperature is high. As we dry off, we begin to feel hot once more.

In cold weather, the skin performs the same pattern in reverse. The pores of the skin remain closed and the heat generated by muscle activity is conserved.

CHAPTER

3

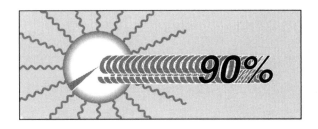

THE SUN:
Cause of over
90% of
Skin
Cancers

*T*here are few of us who don't enjoy a bright sunny day, who don't love a sky dotted with powder-puff clouds. Nonetheless, the sun, so clearly associated with life, warmth, and romance, is now recognized as a prime cause of most skin cancers.

Evidence for the sun's carcinogenic role is unequivocal and overwhelming:

• The more time spent outdoors, the greater the risk of skin cancer. Construction workers, sailors, farmers, and athletes, for example, are at much greater risk of acquiring skin cancer than are people who work indoors.

•Fair-skinned individuals (Irish, Scottish, Scandinavian), who sunburn easily and tan poorly, or minimally, have a higher incidence of skin cancer than brown-skinned individuals (Mexican, African, East Indian), who rarely sunburn but tan profusely.

• In the areas of the United States where the sun is strongest for more hours of the day (such as Southern Arizona, Texas, and Florida), the incidence of skin cancer is proportionately greater than in regions with less sun (Washington, Oregon, Maine).

• Skin cancer rates are higher still in tropical and subtropical regions of the world, where the sun shines more hours of the day and more days of the year. The number of cases of skin cancer in Caucasians increases proportionately the closer one gets to the equator.

• In England, skin cancer occurs more frequently on the right side of the face; in America, it occurs more often on the left. Reason? In England the steering wheel is positioned on the right side of the car—and it is the right side of the face, nearest the open window, that receives the most sun exposure. In America, the situation is reversed.

ULTRAVIOLET RADIATION

What is it about the sun that can cause skin cancer? It isn't the light we can see, but rather the invisible ultraviolet radiation that is the chief culprit: ultraviolet light.

The sunlight we see—visible light—is a very small part of the whole spectrum of electromagnetic radiation emitted by the sun (Figure 3.1). Although we don't usually think of light as radiation, that is exactly what it is. Other forms include x-rays, ultraviolet rays, infrared radiation, microwaves, and even radio waves. These types of radiation are differentiated chiefly by the length of their waves, x-rays being the shortest and radio waves the longest. All wavelengths can penetrate

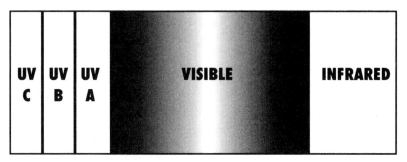

(Figure 3.1) Sunlight spectrum

into the skin to some extent—x-rays penetrate most of all, even through bone.

To indicate how little we see of all the radiation that reaches us: if the entire spectrum were reduced to the height of the book you are now reading, visible light would occupy only a line or so.

The sunlight, or solar radiation, that reaches the earth's surface ranges in wavelength from 290 to 760 nanometers (nm)—a unit of length equivalent to one billionth of a meter.

Visible radiation (400–760 nm) is generally not harmful to normal skin; it cannot tan or burn you. Infrared radiation (over 760 nm) produces the sensation of warmth we feel while in the sunlight. Excessive exposure to infrared can be harmful to the skin.

Ultraviolet radiation can be further subdivided according to its effects on the skin. The longest ultraviolet rays are known as ultraviolet A (UVA) radiation, of wavelengths 320–400 nm. With relatively long exposure (90 minutes or more) UVA light tends to cause tanning and burning. Under normal conditions, however, its capacity to burn the skin is moderate to minimal. But because UVA radiation predominates in the solar energy that reaches the earth's

> 1. **Ultraviolet radiation comprises wavelengths from 290 to 400 nm (UVB 290–320 nm and UVA 320–400 nm)**
> 2. **Visible radiation (wavelengths from 400 to 760 nm)**
> 3. **Infrared radiation (wavelengths longer than 760 nm and up to 3000 nm)**

surface (tenfold to 100-fold more than UVB), it plays a far more important role in contributing to the harmful effects of sun exposure than previously suspected. UVA is known to cause damage to cell membranes and cellular DNA and can contribute to photoaging of the skin as well as the development of skin cancer.

The shorter ultraviolet B (UVB) rays, at 290–320 nm, comprise only two-tenths of 1 percent of all ultraviolet rays we receive. But these short rays are believed to be the primary cause of sunburn, photoaging, and skin cancer. Ultraviolet C (UVC) wavelengths (320–400 nm) from the sun usually do not reach the earth (although exposure to this spectrum can come from other artificial light sources such as germicidal or mercury arc lamps).

FACTORS THAT INFLUENCE SOLAR RADIATION

Season

The sun's intensity varies with the season. In the northern hemisphere, the sun is most intense during the spring, fall, and summer months. It is then that the earth's orbit brings us closest to the sun and the earth tilts toward the sun so that its rays are more direct. In the southern hemisphere, greatest intensity is reached in the fall and winter, for the same reasons.

Time of Day

In the northern hemisphere the sun is strongest during the hours of 10 am to 2 pm (11 am to 3 pm daylight savings time) because the angle of the sun's rays reaching the earth is most direct at these times. As the earth rotates away from the sun, the rays must travel a greater distance before reaching the earth's surface. Thus, as the day passes, the intensity of the sun's rays decreases. In late afternoon and early morning the sun's intensity is only a quarter that of noon.

Latitude

The intensity of the sun's rays increases with proximity to the equator. An inhabitant of an Equatorial country such as Colombia, Kenya, or Indonesia receives dramatically more sunlight than someone living in the United States or Europe.

Those living in the far north—Scandinavian countries, Greenland, or Northern Canada—receive even less than that.

Altitude

The sun's rays increase in intensity approximately 4% for every 300-meter rise in altitude. If you live at a high altitude, or when you are skiing or mountain climbing, sun exposure is markedly increased. In addition, the higher the altitude, the fewer impurities and pollutants there are to block out the damaging ultraviolet radiation. Thus, with respect to skin cancer, people living in smog-ridden cities have a dubious advantage over people living in areas of high altitude and low levels of industrial pollutants.

Climatic and Environmental Conditions

Climate and environmental conditions may markedly affect the amount of sunlight, including damaging ultraviolet radiation, that reaches us. Ultraviolet radiation may be increased by as much as 90%, for example, by reflection off surfaces such as ice, snow, water, or cement.

On overcast or hazy days about 80% of the sun's radiation reaches the earth's surface. Ultraviolet light can cause severe skin damage on such days because infrared rays, which produce the sensation of heat, are filtered by cloud cover. The result is that you feel comfortable and are inclined to stay too long in the sun. In addition, ultraviolet light rays have short wavelengths, bounce off clouds, and hit you from many directions.

The diminishing of the ozone layer, if it continues at current rates, will allow increasing amounts of ultraviolet radiation to penetrate to the earth's surface.

CHAPTER
4

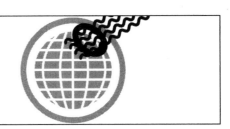

THE
OZONE
CRISIS

Have you ever noticed the sharp, clear, sweet smell in the air after an electrical storm? It is the odor of ozone, a rare, highly unstable form of oxygen that exists in two separate layers: one a very thin layer 10–12 miles above the earth's surface and the other layer at ground level. It is the upper level that absorbs damaging radiation from the sun. If all this ozone were compressed, the band would be no more than 3 mm thick (Figure 4.1).

Ozone composes a tiny but very important part of the earth's atmospheric gases. Very short ultraviolet rays travel from the sun through space until they encounter the outermost layer of the earth's atmosphere. There they convert some of the oxygen present to ozone. The ozone absorbs UVB and, in the process, is reconverted to oxygen. Thus, the ozone layer affords us protection, absorbing all but the 0.2% of all UVB that eventually reaches Earth.

When predictions of the depletion of the ozone layer were first made public in the 1970s, governmental reactions were disbelief and denial, but subsequent studies and data from

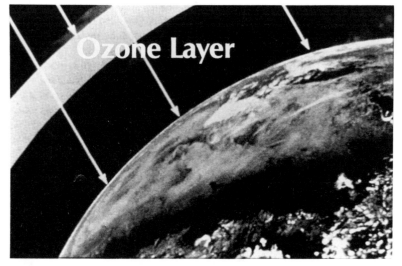

(Figure 4.1) The ozone layer, a thin band of the earth's atmospheric gas that filters out much of the sun's dangerous ultraviolet radiation, is diminishing rapidly; therefore, more ultraviolet rays are bombarding us.

satellites confirmed the reports. By 1985, the National Academy of Science affirmed that for several months during each year, as much as 50% of the ozone layer is depleted over Halley Bay, Antarctica—a hole in the ozone layer the size of Canada, and growing larger.

A 5% decrease in the ozone layer in other parts of the world, which scientists believe is likely, will result in a 10% increase in biologically effective radiation. Populations experiencing this additional radiation over the next 20 years would be afflicted with epidemic increases in skin cancer: for melanoma, 5%–8%; for basal cell carcinoma, as much as 10%; and for squamous cell carcinoma, as much as 20%. Thus, the fragile balance that maintains the ozone layer, increasingly threatened, is of critical importance to us all (Figure 4.2).

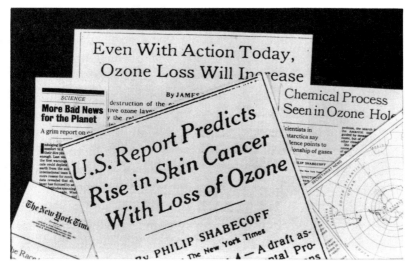

(Figure 4.2) The greatest hazard humans face from the effects of ozone depletion is skin cancer, which is increasing at an alarming rate.

The studies conducted in the 1970s implicated chlorofluorocarbons as the agents causing the depletion of ozone. These chemicals were introduced commercially to replace ammonia, CO_2, and hydrocarbons as refrigerants. The chemicals were subsequently used in countless products, at first mainly as spray propellants in paints, solvents, cleaners, coolants, deodorants, hairsprays, shaving creams, toppings, etc. (In 1973, more than 3 billion spray cans were marketed in the United States—14 for every inhabitant.) Subsequently, the United States banned most of these uses. However, chlorofluorocarbons then became widely used as cleansers in the computer industry and in the manufacture of foam insulation, packaging, and padding inserts.

Ironically, at first the chemicals seemed ideal: light, chemically inert, nonflammable, nontoxic, noncarcinogenic, noncorrosive, and highly energy efficient. They were considered harmless to the environment. Their very inertness, however, allows them to reach the upper atmosphere without being destroyed. There, the more intense solar radiation frees the chlorine, which combines with ozone to create chlorine oxide. In turn, this forms diatomic oxygen, causing progressive destruction of the ozone layer.

Although the use of chlorofluorocarbon (CFC) in spray propellants has been banned for the present in the United States, the growth in demand for other uses has led to continued increases in production. Moreover, other nations have continued to manufacture and use CFCs in aerosols as well as a variety of other products. Concern for the potential effects of the continued use of CFCs has led the United States to join with a large number of other industrialized nations to develop controls on CFC production. Originally, the plan was to drop to 50% of 1986 production levels by 1992. Recent evidence suggests that even this will not be enough and new negotiations are under way that call for a complete phaseout. Substitute chemicals known as hydrochlorofluorocarbons (HFCs), though less damaging to the ozone layer than CFCs, also pose a threat, and efforts to restore the ozone layer call for controls on these propellants as well as a phaseout of halons and methyl chloroform.

5

DYING FOR A TAN: No Tan Is a Safe Tan

Many of us regard the stinging redness that results from our first summer outing as a mild and temporary discomfort, a small price to pay for the coppery "good looks" that will soon be ours. We smear on more oil, hold up our metal reflectors, and turn ourselves slowly, baking our skins—roasts on a spit.

Tell me, would you hold your unprotected hand over a flame—even for a second? Probably not. And yet, in tanning yourself, that's exactly what you are doing. The effects of sun exposure are nearly all detrimental. The momentary pain of a sunburn is the least of it. Premature aging, eye damage, and, of even greater consequence, skin cancer can all result. You may be, quite literally, dying for a tan.

THE "SUNSHINE VITAMIN"—How Much Do You Need?

But, you may be thinking, don't we need some sunlight for our health? Vitamin D has long been known as the "sunshine" vitamin. Exposed to the ultraviolet rays from the sun, our bodies can convert a vitamin D precursor located in the skin into active vitamin D itself. This vitamin D is essential for calcium and phosphate metabolism in the formation and repair of bones. Without sunshine, this process does not occur. Fifty years ago, the rule was "the more sunshine, the better." Now we know that about 10–15 minutes of sun exposure a day are needed to obtain adequate vitamin D, especially in the United States, where our diets are rich in vitamin D-containing foods such as milk, eggs, and butter. In addition, many products are now "fortified" with additional vitamin D.

Vitamin D deficiency can cause rickets, a softening of bony tissue, and dental caries (cavities). Blacks are somewhat more susceptible to the disease because melanin pigment absorbs ultraviolet radiation, preventing it from reaching the skin's deeper layers where vitamin D precursors are located. Similarly, a poorly nourished individual confined indoors for extended periods of time might be at risk. In practice, though, vitamin D deficiency is rare in the United States today and easily avoided through a proper diet.

WHEN SUN STRIKES SKIN: TANNING AND BURNING

Many of us think that sunburns and suntans are part of the same process—"I got really burned, but then it faded into a tan." "Some people just have to burn first if they want to get a good tan." In fact, although burns and tans are caused by the same kinds of ultraviolet radiation, and both represent sun damage, they are largely distinct processes.

The longer ultraviolet A (UVA) rays are capable of tanning

the skin without producing a burn (although exposure to huge amounts of UVA radiation—60–90 minutes of midday sun, or about 30 minutes under an artificial tanning lamp—can also burn). These rays penetrate deep into the dermis and stimulate melanin production.

Shorter ultraviolet B (UVB) rays also stimulate the tanning reaction, and aı ; the chief cause of sunburn and skin cancer. (If you have trouble remembering which is which, remember that B of UVB rays stands for "burning" of the skin!) These rays initially affect and damage the epidermal (outer) layer of the skin. They are absorbed largely by cells located there, and both sunburn and skin cancer are to a great extent conditions that start in the epidermis.

Ultraviolet light falling on the skin is selectively absorbed by melanin (dark skin absorbs radiation more readily than does light skin). Dark skin thus enjoys special protection against the sun, possibly because the "soaking up" of UVB by melanin means that less radiation is absorbed by the rest of the epidermis, specifically basal and squamous cells, which appear to be especially vulnerable to damage from ultraviolet radiation.

Tanning

When sunlight strikes skin, a sequence of protective reactions is initiated, probably triggered by exposure to UVA and UVB radiation. This "tanning response" occurs in three stages. First, preexisting melanin granules close to the surface of the skin are oxidized, causing them to darken. This is usually initiated by UVA. Next, melanocytes located somewhat deeper are stimulated to produce and transfer new pigment granules to the uppermost levels of the skin, for additional protection—like an army bringing in its reserves. Finally, a cell-dividing impulse allows the pigment cells to proliferate and to produce more melanin, a process that takes from 5 to 7 days.

Melanin production is determined genetically. Dark-skinned persons have naturally pigmented skins as well as the capacity to produce a lot more melanin, should they need to do so. Fair-skinned peop e, on the other hand, have little pigmentation in their skins and little capacity to produce more melanin. Thus they are essentially defenseless against ultraviolet radiation. Fair-skinned people should keep in mind that tanning is predetermined genetically. They will tan just so much and no more, no matter how long they stay in the sun.

It is important to remember that tanning is the body's natural, biologic response to the harmful rays of the sun. In other words, when a tan begins, some damage has already been done. There is no such thing as "a safe tan."

Sunburn

Skin that is sunburned has been damaged by ultraviolet radiation (chiefly UVB radiation). A mild sunburn looks red because the vessels close to the surface of the skin are injured and swollen. This skin reddening, called erythema, may begin after only a few minutes of exposure, but it may continue to worsen for 24–72 hours, depending upon the duration of sun exposure.

REPEATED SUN EXPOSURE: THE DAMAGE ADDS UP

Some time after a sunburn or a suntan, the skin appears to go "back to normal," looking as if the sun-induced change had disappeared completely. Nothing could be further from the truth. The cellular damage caused by ultraviolet radiation is cumulative and often irreversible (Figure 5.1). I see the evidence each day in my office: dryness, wrinkling, splotches of pigmentation, thickening and sagging, and, often, precancerous growths or skin cancer itself.

I like to compare the process of sun-induced skin damage to that of cooking an egg. If you dip a raw egg in boiling water it profoundly changes the proteins, causing them to become cooked—eventually a hard-boiled egg.

Given enough sun exposure, anyone, with any skin coloration, can experience cosmetic damage and skin cancer; however, these conditions are more prevalent in fair-skinned

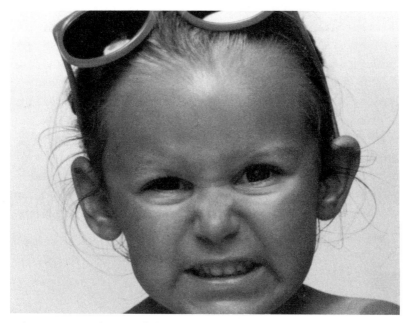

(Figure 5.1) A history of blistering sunburns in childhood increases your risk of developing skin cancer.

individuals. Albinos, who genetically lack the capacity to produce melanin, are deprived entirely of a natural sun shield.

On a small island in Honduras, there is an Indian tribe of albinos, called "moon children," who go outside mostly at night because they can't tolerate the intense sunburns they experience during the day. Despite their nocturnal life, they often live only a brief 20 years before they die of skin cancer.

PHOTOSENSITIVITY REACTIONS

There is a separate but related cause of sun damage that appears to result more from UVA than from UVB rays. These are photosensitivity reactions, which can be induced by medicated soaps and perfumes, and even by medications (antibiotics, oral contraceptives, diuretics, tranquilizers, antidiabetic agents, and antihistamines). These drugs can absorb the energy in sunlight to form biologically reactive molecules that subsequently lead to skin reactions. Symptoms of these skin reactions include rashes, blistering, and an erythema that is both painful and prolonged. There is generally no special history of skin cancer with such patients.

6

SUN
SUSCEPTIBILITY:
Determining
Your
Danger
Point

Now that you are aware of the dangers of too much sun, I can almost hear your next question. Is there a sensible way to enjoy the outdoors and still have healthy skin? The answer is yes—if you take a few precautions. The most important precaution is to avoid the sun's ultraviolet rays; just how to do this will be discussed later on in this chapter and in subsequent ones.

Your first step should be determining your own personal susceptibility to the sun. You'll want to take into consideration your skin type, elements of your health history, how quickly you burn, and how much of a "sun worshipper" you are. This information will tell you how much sun protection you need to lessen your chance of getting skin cancer.

WHAT'S MY SKIN TYPE

The degree to which a person tans or sunburns depends on genetic factors and on the natural pigmentation of the skin. Six skin types are designated, ranked from skin type I, the most sun-sensitive, to skin type VI, the least vulnerable to sun damage (Table 1 and Figure 6.1).

In deciding on your skin type, give careful thought to your medical history, especially your history of tanning and burning. Sometimes, a person may look like a skin type III but have a history of frequent burning that designates him as a type II. If you are not sure, place yourself in a higher category rather than a lower one.

TABLE 1: KNOW YOUR SKIN TYPE

Skin Type	Skin Reactions	Examples
I	Always burns easily and severely (painful burn); tans little or not at all and peels.	People with fair skin, blue or even brown eyes, freckles; unexposed skin is white.
II	Usually burns easily and severely (painful burn); tans minimally or lightly, also peels.	People with fair skin, red, blond or brown hair, blue, hazel or brown eyes; unexposed skin is white.
III	Burns moderately, tans about average.	Average Caucasian; unexposed skin is white.
IV	Burns minimally; tans easily and above average with each exposure; exhibits IPD* reaction.	People with white or light brown skin, dark brown hair, dark eyes; unexposed skin is white or light brown.
V	Rarely burns, tans easily and substantially; always exhibits IPD* reaction.	Brown-skinned persons; unexposed skin is brown.
VI	Never burns and tans profusely; exhibits IPD* reaction.	Black persons; unexposed skin is black.

*IPD Immediate Pigment Darkening

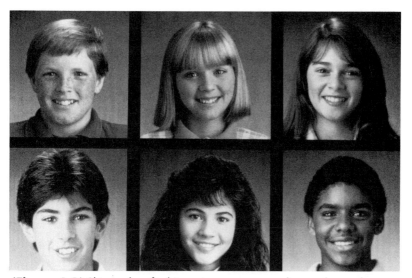

(Figure 6.1) Skin is classified into six groups according to the tendency to sunburn.

Factors in your health history that place you at higher risk for skin cancer—and mandate extra protection—include: a family history of skin cancer, a personal history of skin cancer, a record of painful or blistering sunburns, especially when young, and any precancerous lesions.

Minimal Erythema Dose

Minimal erythema dose (MED) is a convenient way to quantify sun damage. It is defined as "the smallest amount of sunlight exposure necessary to induce a barely perceptible redness of the skin within 24 hours after sun exposure" (the medical term for this redness is erythema). Knowing your usual MED gives you a good idea of how much sun you can be exposed to with relatively low risk and is determined by your personal sun susceptibility and by environmental conditions that influence sun intensity.

Because erythema signals that damage has already been done, 1 MED is over the maximum that a person should receive; the goal of a sun protection program is to stay well under this amount each day.

A variety of environmental and climatic conditions influence sun intensity (and with it, the MED). During any one day, for example, intensity of the sun varies significantly. Some newspapers routinely report the sun intensity index, an estimate of minutes in the sun required to redden average, untanned skin based on the daily weather forecast. A sample of these predictions for an average, untanned Caucasian on a typical day in Arizona is given in Table 2.

TABLE 2: MED CALCULATIONS
Time Required for 1 MED

Hour	Minutes
9:00 am	54
10:00 am	29
11:00 am	20
noon	17
1:00 pm	15
2:00 pm	16
3:00 pm	20
4:00 pm	33

This same average, untanned white person standing not in Tucson but in far northern Barrow, Alaska, on the same day would take far longer to accumulate 1 MED. Less time would be required close to the Equator in Panama.

In like manner, an unusually fair-skinned person in Tucson at noon might accumulate 1 MED in only 10 minutes, while a dark-skinned individual standing beside him would require half an hour for the same amount of damage to take place. The most MEDs anyone could accumulate in the Northern hemisphere are approximately 15 MEDs of UVB and about 4 MEDs of UVA. A fair-skinned person standing near the equator on a clear, bright summer day from 9 am to 4 pm would accumulate about this amount (as well as a very severe sunburn!).

To determine your sun sensitivity, expose the inner part of your forearm to about 15 minutes of sun on a clear, sunny summer day at noon, and check exposed areas. If any reddening appears—immediately or by the next day—you are a very sun-sensitive individual and must exert all possible precautions against the sun. If no reddening is visible you can allow yourself to remain in the sun a little bit longer the next day.

Although your precise MED will differ somewhat with time and environmental conditions, knowing your usual noontime MED gives you a good idea of how much sun protection you need. The average MED for an untanned white person (who is not wearing any kind of sunscreen or sunblock) at noon is about 15–20 minutes. The MED can be approximately doubled to 30 minutes if the person is in a shaded area. (Remember—ultraviolet radiation penetrates materials and bounces off objects, so even in the shade you aren't fully protected!)

SUN AFFINITY RATIO

Next, try to establish your sun affinity ratio (SAR) or sun-seeking behavior, the amount of time you actually spend in the sun. The SAR is an estimate of the average number of hours (or minutes) spent outdoors per day, all year-round. So often, patients with visible sun damage tell me that they spend virtually no time in the sun. How can persons who haven't been exposed to the sun have sun-damaged skins? They can't. Skin is damaged like this only by being exposed to radiation—either from the sun itself or from sunlamps and tanning booths.

When my patients tell me they spend almost no time in the sun, they may mean that they spend no *intentional* time tanning at the beach. Yet sun-exposed skin tans or burns just as easily when you play softball, hike, ski, or perform outdoor chores as it does when you sun yourself at the beach. Don't forget driving, walking those five blocks from the train to the office, walking your dog, and chatting on the sidewalk with a friend or neighbor. All of these constitute "sun time."

SAR alone is a good predictor of future skin cancer. For persons with a high SAR who use no sunscreen the likelihood of developing skin cancer is frighteningly high: for men, 26,999 skin cancer cases per 100,000 population by age 55; for women, 26,254 skin cancer cases per 100,000 population by age 55. For persons with a low SAR, who practice sun avoidance, the contrast in incidence of skin cancer is striking: for men, 1,614 per 100,000; for women, approximately 900 per 100,000—a drastic reduction.

USING THE INFORMATION: SUNSCREENS AND SPF

Once you've determined your skin type, MED, and SAR,

you should have a good idea of how much sun protection you need. The elements are additive: if you are a skin type I or II, are frequently in the sun, and accumulate 1 MED in less time than it takes the average person, you are at high risk and need all the protection you can get. If you are an adult, you have probably already damaged your skin significantly during childhood and need to be extraordinarily cautious. A darker-skinned person living in a northern region who works in an office and spends most of his or her free time indoors is not at such high risk. (Unfortunately, we cannot say this person is at no risk, or even low risk, because other elements contribute to the development of skin cancer.)

Sunscreens are currently the best protection against ultraviolet rays. Many products on the market today filter out both UVA and UVB. Generous and frequent application of effective sunscreens lowers the risk of sun-induced wrinkling, premature aging, and skin cancer.

The Sun Protection Factor (SPF) is a number used to indicate the effectiveness of a sunscreen in preventing erythema, or redness. The SPF of the sunscreen is MED with a sunscreen divided by MED without a sunscreen:

$$SPF = \frac{\text{MED of sunscreen-protected skin}}{\text{MED of unprotected skin}}$$

Thus, if unprotected skin showed erythema following 30 minutes of exposure and the skin protected by sunscreen was red after 7½ hours of exposure, the SPF of the sunscreen would be 15. In other words, the protected skin would require 15 times as long (or a dose of UVR 15 times as large) to develop erythema.

The United States Food and Drug Administration (FDA) has designated the following categories for labelling of sunscreen products:

CATEGORY OF SUNSCREEN PRODUCT

SPF

Minimal sun protection **2–4**

Moderate sun protection. **4–6**

Extra sun protection **6–8**

Maximal. **8–15**

Ultra. .... **15+**

Using a sunscreen with too little protection can obviously be dangerous. If your usual MED is 30 minutes and you wear a sunscreen of SPF 8, you will accumulate 1 MED in approximately 4.5 hours. That may be adequate if you plan to play tennis for 2 or 3 hours. On the other hand, if your MED is 15 minutes and you use a sunscreen of 4, you'll reach 1 MED in only 1 hour—hardly enough for a day hiking in the mountains! I strongly recommend a sunscreen with an SPF of 15 or greater for everyone; the extra protection makes good sun sense and will give you real peace of mind.

CHAPTER

7

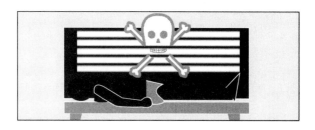

ARTIFICIAL SUN: Sunlamps and Tanning Booths

Deep in the wintertime, do you seek out a booth in your local "health" club or tanning salon to try to recapture last summer's deep, dark glow? Tanning booths have grown greatly in popularity in the past 5 years. But sunlamps, whether used at home or in a tanning booth, offer no therapeutic benefit. You may feel a transient psychological lift from the warmth and relaxation or from your "improved cosmetic appearance," but your skin and general health are being assaulted (Figure 7.1). Unless you are under medical treatment for certain skin conditions that make use of ultraviolet light (always under strict supervision of a physician), there is no good reason to use a sunlamp.

PARLOR OPERATORS: "SUNLAMPS ARE SAFE!"

We performed a telephone survey of seven tanning salons in our immediate neighborhood, asking questions regarding type of equipment, type of ultraviolet radiation, required or advised number of visits, length of visit and exposure, and

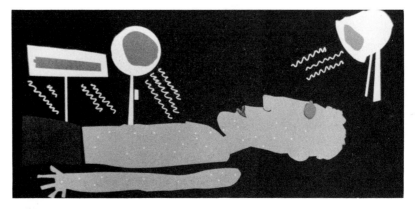

(Figure 7.1) The "safe" tan promised you by many tanning salons simply does not exist.

sunscreen and eyewear (protective goggles) use. What did we find? Tanning salon operators often promote their establishments as safe—in marked contrast to the opinion of medical experts.

All respondents answered willingly. Some were operators and some were employees. The first question, "is tanning in a booth safer for my skin?" drew the following replies:

"Safer than the sun!"

"Nobody's ever been burned."

"You can do it every day of the week if you want. Sure it's safe. Unlimited."

"Oh yes, these lights can't burn you. Of course, you shouldn't overdo it—three or four times a week is okay."

Only one operator hesitated a bit, then said, "Well, some doctors say you shouldn't get any tan, but if you want one, these lights are okay, not detrimental." This last respondent also suggested that some skin types did not tan easily in the sun or in the booth. "Once you get a base tan, though, it's easy to maintain."

All respondents assured the questioner that their equipment was the best, most recent, and safest available. The lights were described variously as "bulbs," "tanning lamps," "UVA lights," and "quartz lights." One stated the lights were "made in Germany" as though that validated them. Another described the lights for a tube bed ("we call it a coffin bed...") as mercury lamps with a phosphorus coating. "That way more UVB gets through, but they're still safe."

The beds were usually made of acrylic, some cushioned, some concave. Some required that the occupant turn after 20 minutes from the front to the back, because the lamps radiated only from above. Others had lamps both above and directly below the acrylic sheet—as many as 24 bulbs, so that no turning was necessary. In two salons, face machines were available for head and chest exposure only.

The respondents mentioned UVA and UVB but without much assurance and with little clarity. Three said their salons used lights with between 98% and 99% UVA and only 1%–2% UVB.

"UVB is what causes skin cancer, you know," said one. "UVB. That's the bad stuff. UVB is what will burn you. UVA only tans. We have 2% UVB because you need to activate the melanin pigment, but that's not enough to hurt you."

One said that he had listened to a researcher on a TV program who had pronounced as safe the type of lights used in his salon, "But then he got too scientific and I couldn't follow him." Another said that the sun "is 90% UVB, so we limit UVB." All assured the questioner that there was no remote possibility of skin damage, far less of skin cancer.

Most respondents recommended three or four visits during the initial week, and some suggested up to five. Every one of them mentioned the need for a "base tan." Some suggested three days of tanning in a row with one day of no tanning, followed by three more. All said that regular visits were required weekly thereafter, with as many as seven visits a week to as few as one or two. Limits for exposure from 20 to 40 minutes per visit were advised.

Respondents were all emphatic about the use of sunscreens.

"Can't use a sun block. That would defeat the whole purpose."

"No sunscreen. There's no need for one."

Instead, all salon operators or employees said they sold a lotion, described as an activator or stimulator of tanning reaction or as a moisturizer, in case of dryness, to be used after the tanning session.

"It will intensify your tan."

All but one respondent said they offered and recommended use of goggles. One specified that goggles in use in his salon were FDA approved and that patrons should not keep their eyes open or attempt to read or watch television while under tanning lamps. The one operator who did not suggest goggles said, "You can just keep your eyes closed." The cost quoted for the dubious pleasure was not high in any of the salons, ranging from $.10 per minute for a tube bed with mercury lights; $.20 a minute for quartz lights; a month of daily sessions for $19.00; 10 sessions a month for $25.00 (with two free sessions); to $12.00 per session. "A lot cheaper than a week in the Islands," volunteered the operator of this last salon.

Pretty cheap?

If you think so, your tan can cost you much more than 10 cents a minute. It may cost you your appearance and even your life. The "coffin bed" may be a more appropriate term than the operator realized.

THE MEDICAL POINT OF VIEW: "TANNING SPELLS TROUBLE"

According to The Skin Cancer Foundation and other reputable scientific authorities, exposure to the radiation of a tanning booth may be more risky than exposure to the sun. We really know very little about their long-term effects, but we do know that severe burns can result when sunlamps are used without caution. Operators may be self-serving or negligent; employees may be transient or ignorant of potential dangers.

And because the industry is virtually unregulated, there are no standards or supervision of equipment and procedures.

Sunlamps have many hazards. First, let us consider the "safety" of the ultraviolet A, the major component of the ultraviolet radiation that is emitted in tanning booths and that is advocated by their operators as harmless, even beneficial.

Ultraviolet A affects the deeper layers of the skin, causing direct injury to blood vessels. It can cause collagen breakdown, reducing skin elasticity; inflammation of the stratum corneum; and increased pigmentation (melanin deposition) in the deeper layers of the skin. It can also damage the eye, and more importantly, results in decreased amounts of Langerhans' cells, vital immunologic cells found in the epidermis and necessary for the body's defense. In addition, UVA augments the damage produced by ultraviolet B. Finally, recent scientific evidence suggests that prolonged exposure to ultraviolet A alone can in itself cause skin cancer.

The lights found in tanning parlors frequently emit UVB

radiation as well as UVA; the intensity of UVB light emitted by one lamp we measured was as strong as the summer sunlight at noon in New York!

One of the greatest hazards of combined UVA/UVB is burning of the cornea of the eye. Prolonged exposure to ultraviolet radiation without adequate protection can result in irrevocable retinal damage and/or cataracts. Any eye irritation caused by sunlamps requires prompt treatment by an ophthalmologist. Corneal burns must be treated with antibiotic ointments, and the eye should be covered until healing occurs—about 72 hours. Proper eye covering—protective, polarized goggles—should be worn whenever you are exposed to sunlamps.

REGULATIONS FOR PARLORS

Recognizing the dangers, states have begun to pass laws regulating tanning salons. A law recently enacted in Texas requires that people 18 or younger must show written permission from a parent or guardian before they can use commercial tanning devices, and those under age 14 must be accompanied by a parent or guardian. In addition, all customers must sign a written agreement acknowledging the risks of overexposure and agreeing to use protective eyewear. The FDA prohibits salon owners from promoting tanning booths as free from risk. The only claim permitted for indoor tanning devices is that of "cosmetic tanning." Some states have enacted or are considering legislation to regulate tanning facilities.

The tanning industry is difficult to monitor. Parlors and booths spring up and disappear overnight, often as adjuncts to beauty parlors and hair salons, health clubs, and spas. Until more rigid regulations are in place, it is up to you, the consumer, to protect yourself.

HOW TO PROTECT YOURSELF

If you do choose to patronize tanning parlors, minimize the damage by taking the following steps.

First, ask questions about the types of lights and equipment used. Be sure that the booths have both timers and attendants. Verify that proper protective goggles are provided and be sure to wear them.

Be suspicious if no questions are asked of you, particularly with regard to skin type, medical conditions, and current medications; sensitivities or allergies; previous skin cancer or treatment with UV light for psoriasis, and prior x-ray therapy for acne.

Use a sunscreen. You will tan more slowly, but you will decrease damage. If an operator attempts to persuade you that tanning is completely without hazard or advises against using a sunscreen, go elsewhere.

Better still, don't do it at all.

CHAPTER

8

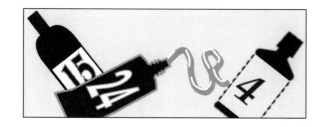

SUN BLOCKERS, SUNSCREENS, and Other Effective Agents

While 50 years ago fashionable ladies carried parasols and wore long-sleeved dresses and gloves to protect themselves from the sun, today's methods of sun protection are far more effective and convenient. Materials—clothing, hats, beach umbrellas, and the like—still have their place. But in addition, today we have physical and chemical sunshields; the most important of these, sunscreens, can be thought of as your "second skin."

But beware. Also on the market are a number of ineffective or even dangerous products that manufacturers claim can help you tan or protect you from the sun. Suntan lotions and tanning pills are numbered in this group.

CLOTHING AND OTHER MATERIALS

Clothing is such a natural part of our daily lives that we may not think of it as sun protection. But it does help shield us from ultraviolet light. Don't overlook its value. In the workaday world, wear a hat to help protect your ears and any bald spots up top. At the beach, your main shield will be a sunscreen, but after that game of volleyball or that refreshing swim, stay under a beach umbrella and wear a terrycloth robe, pants, and long sleeves. Don't forget a good pair of polarized sunglasses and a hat. All these items can minimize your exposure to ultraviolet radiation (Figure 8.1).

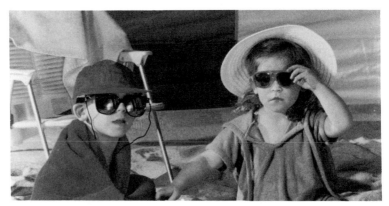

(Figure 8.1) Always wear protective clothing such as broadbrimmed hats, polarized sunglasses, long sleeves, and pants.

SUN BLOCKERS: REFLECTORS OF ULTRAVIOLET B

Sun blockers are physical agents that reflect and scatter ultraviolet rays. These products include formulations containing titanium dioxide, zinc oxide, kaolin, talc, or iron oxide.

They are invariably effective and spread easily over the skin. However, they have a number of serious disadvantages. They wash off easily, are unsightly, messy, impractical for covering large areas of skin, and when worn at the beach their stickiness allows sand to adhere to the skin. Some of these products can cause stinging and are irritants, especially to the eyes. Also, some will temporarily discolor clothing. They may cause worsening of skin conditions such as folliculitis (inflammation of the hair follicles) or whiteheads, because they tend to block the pores of the skin.

Opaque sunblocks are excellent, however, for applying on the nose and rims of the ears during outdoor activity in strong sunlight. They also may be the sun protection of choice for persons who suffer from melasma — hyperpigmentation that results in brown spots or blotches, or for women who are pregnant or take oral contraceptives.

SUNSCREENS: CHEMICAL ABSORBERS OF ULTRAVIOLET RADIATION

A sunscreen is a chemically formulated product applied to the skin that absorbs, rather than reflects, the sun's ultraviolet rays, thus protecting the skin in a manner similar to the natural pigment melanin.

Sunscreens are developed and tested with the aid of special lamps called solar simulators. Solar simulators produce light with a spectrum similar to that of sunlight, but without interference from other factors like season, latitude, moisture, time of day, or dust in the air. This permits investigators to quantify the protection afforded by the sunscreen based on exposure to a known quantity of ultraviolet radiation simulating sunlight. However, interfering factors are not accounted for, so you must remember to take them into consideration yourself. A sunscreen can be formulated to protect against UVA rays, UVB rays, or both.

Basic chemical categories of sunscreens are: PABA (para-aminobenzoic acid), PABA esters, benzophenones, cinnamates, and anthranilates. (A list of approved sunscreens is available from The Skin Cancer Foundation, Box 561, New York, NY 10156.) Sunscreens may be formulated in alcohols, gels, oils, butters, balms, or aerosols; cosmetic appearance is quite acceptable.

Not all sunscreens offer complete protection. Persons with skin types I and II may burn if they indulge in excessive sunbathing no matter what product they use; they should not expose themselves to the sun for long periods in search of an elusive tan. Similarly, persons with skin types III and IV will almost always experience some degree of tanning despite application of sunscreen with a high SPF. So far, the sun and your genetic makeup predominate over any sunscreen.

SUNSCREEN INGREDIENTS

PABA

PABA sunscreens, some of the earliest effective sunscreens, absorb and filter UVB. However, because of their high alcohol content, these early sunscreens washed off easily and were difficult to apply uniformly. They had to be frequently reapplied, and caused some minor skin irritation. They also caused temporary discoloration of clothing from photooxidation.

A new generation of PABA came into being a few years ago. The new and improved sunscreens employ PABA esters, which attach themselves to the stratum corneum, the outer layer of the skin, and are so water-resistant that they can resist 40–80 minutes of whirlpool washing and still retain over 50% of their effectiveness. A combination of these esters can also extend the protective range further, to the UVA spectrum, and residual absorption of these esters in the stratum corneum offers some further protection. Such combinations are now the most commonly used sunscreens. To date, more than 21 different chemicals have been approved for use by the FDA.

Cinnamates

Cinnamate sunscreens have an SPF of 15 and provide protection in the UVB range (290–320 nm). Although they are generally effective, they may cause contact dermatitis, especially in persons who are sensitive to products containing cinnamon.

Benzophenones

Sunscreens containing benzophenone absorb and scatter UVA. Although not as effective against UVB unless they contain two or more active sunscreen chemicals, they provide good protection in snow, high altitudes, and against reflected light. When used in combination with PABA esters, they are effective in areas of high humidity because they do not wash off easily.

Anthranilates

Anthranilate sunscreens provide moderate protection against both UVA and UVB.

COMBINATION AGENTS

Many sunscreens on the market are combinations of several of the above agents. Sunscreens containing combinations of benzophenones or cinnamates provide good protection against drug-induced photosensitivity reactions. Agents containing mainly UVB absorbers with less potent UVA absorbers will allow some tanning. Combinations of benzophenones and Padimate-O (Escalol 507) are also usually effective in preventing sunburn reactions during prolonged exposure to solar radiation or in preventing drug-induced phototoxic reactions.

"HIGH-OCTANE" SUNSCREENS

The introduction of the newest "super" sunscreens that have an SPF of 20–30 and higher originally started mainly as a marketing ploy. One might believe that 15—which I recommend—is good, 20 is better, and 30 the best. Hypothetically speaking, in this world it would be difficult to find a place where even the fairest-skinned individual could accumulate ultraviolet exposure of more than 15 MEDs. For this reason, I did not believe the "super" sunscreens offered any advantage. Now the thinking is changing. There may be some extra protection for those with sensitive skin, patients with a history of skin cancer, or anyone who puts on the sunscreen too thinly. Recent clinical studies have shown that people tend to apply much less sunscreen (about one-half the amount) per square inch than is used in the testing which determines the SPF rating of a sunscreen. Furthermore, the SPF values measured in the laboratory are considerably higher than those reported for actual use of the same products in sunlight. Also, for people who swim or sweat, sunscreen may be diluted or wiped off. Consequently, our recommendation is at minimum SPF 15; higher numbers if you like them and find them beneficial.

CHOOSING A SUNSCREEN

You will want a sunscreen that looks good, and that feels and smells good to you. An excellent choice for daily protection is a sunscreen-containing makeup.

There are many sunscreens on the market with sun protection factors (SPF) ranging from a low of 2 to a high of over 50. The sunscreen best suited to your needs depends on several indications, but particularly on your skin type and your MED.

SPF #15 or Higher
Sun
Protection
Factor

I recommend maximum protection for everyone—an SPF of no less than 15 that filters UVA and UVB. Some other authorities would adopt more latitude, recommending an SPF of 15 for skin types I and II, but allowing 10–15 for skin type III, an 8–10 for skin type IV, a 6–8 for skin type V, and a 4–6 for skin type VI. In my opinion, these would provide only minimal coverage though they are better than no sunscreen at all.

When you choose your sunscreen, remember all that you have learned about environmental factors such as altitude and reflection from snow, sand, or water. Also, the longer your exposure to the sun, either for recreation or by occupation, the more you need a sunscreen. You may want to have on hand sunscreens of different strengths—use an SPF 15 for tennis or hiking for several hours in the summertime while an SPF 6, or a sunscreen-containing makeup, will do for daily wear when sun exposure is limited to mornings and evenings.

Other qualities to look for are substantivity and water-resistance. I use the term substantivity to describe a sunscreen that exhibits persistence and adheres well to the skin; it combines with the outer layer of the skin and retains good protective effect after the wearer sweats or swims. The PABA ester family falls into this category, especially if these sunscreens are applied one-half hour to 1 hour prior to sun exposure. The water-resistant and waterproof property is a recent marketing term denoting that a product has been tested for a period of 40–80 minutes of swimming or water immersion while maintaining effective protection. These are ideal for athletes—swimmers, joggers—or others who perspire during outdoor activity.

PRECAUTIONS

Several other factors must be taken into consideration when choosing your sunscreen. These include your state of health, any skin conditions, either current or chronic, and any concurrent medication or treatment you take. Also, many cosmetics, dyes, sprays, and perfumes may interact with ingredients used in sunscreens. Your physician or pharmacist can advise you.

Persons with very sensitive or irritated skin should not use a product with an alcohol base. PABA esters can cause contact dermatitis (or inflammation) on sensitive skin or photodermatitis (a light-stimulated dermatitis that appears some time after the product is applied).

In some products, antioxidants are added as preservatives.

Other products contain cocoa butter or almond oil. These ingredients may combine to cause a reaction in persons taking certain medications or using other cosmetics, perfumes, coloring agents, or hair dyes.

You can perform a quick and simple test, known as a "patch test," to determine your sensitivity to any sunscreen: apply a small amount of a sunscreen to a test area the size of a nickel on the inside of your upper arm; cover the patch with an adhesive bandage and observe the spot a few hours later and again 24 hours later. If you notice any redness or itching, do not use the product.

Finally, look for the Seal of Recommendation of The Skin Cancer Foundation, an acceptance awarded to a number of products with an SPF of 15 or greater that meet the stringent criteria of the Foundation's Photobiology Committee.

APPLICATION AND USE

Should a sunscreen be used every day? The answer depends on who you are, the time of year, and your occupation. In the wintertime, if you are simply walking across the street in the late afternoon, I don't believe it is necessary, even for someone with a history of skin cancer. But if you are going to spend half an hour outdoors in the afternoon of that same day, it would be wise to apply sunscreen before going outside (Figure 8.2). In spring, fall, and summer it is wise to make sunscreen use routine—apply it every morning, with the same regularity with which you brush your teeth. If you work outdoors, reapply frequently during the day; for office workers, one morning application should be sufficient.

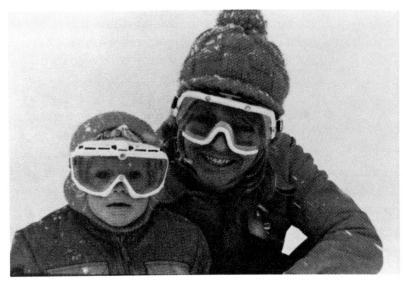

(Figure 8.2) You should use a sunscreen in the winter when spending time outdoors because the sun's rays reflect off the snow.

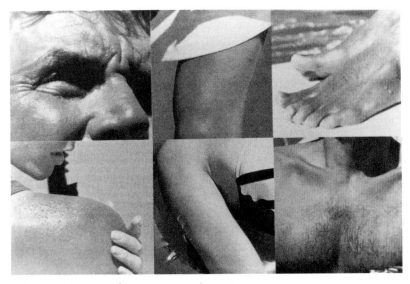

(Figure 8.3) Don't forget to cover these six sun-sensitive areas.

No sunscreen is effective unless it is applied properly. Use it as follows:

1. Apply the sunscreen carefully to all areas of skin that will be exposed to the sun at least 15–30 minutes before you go outdoors. Pay attention to areas that are often neglected, such as earlobes, neck, lips, nose, and bald spots (Figure 8.3).

2. Reapply it frequently and liberally at least every two hours as long as you are in the sun's rays, being sure that no spots are left uncovered. Swimming, perspiring heavily, and exposure to strong winds call for more frequent reapplication of the product you choose.

3. Use a water-resistant sunscreen and one with an SPF slightly higher than you think you need. The Skin Cancer Foundation recommends use of high-protection sunscreens—15 or greater—at all times.

This advice about sunscreens applies to all skin types and all ages. The fact that your skin is dark or tends to tan does not mean that you can't get skin cancer.

INEFFECTIVE OR DANGEROUS SUN PRODUCTS

"Suntan" Lotions

For many years people have used a multitude of substances in the hope of preventing sunburn while at the same time acquiring a tan; some of these substances include mineral oil, cooking oil, olive oil, cocoa butter, and iodine. Commercial tanning lotions and creams promise a deep tan, but instead of assisting the tanning process they merely oil or lubricate the skin. This allows ultraviolet radiation to penetrate with greater strength and to deeper skin layers, causing damage.

Tanning Pills

Researchers are developing and testing sunscreen pills in the search for a safe, effective product that can be taken by mouth. A few are already in use as prescription drugs by persons with health problems or skin conditions that require special treatment or that prevent them from using topical sunscreens.

Among the agents tested or currently in use are beta-carotene, chloroquine, and oxsoralen (methoxsalen or 8-methoxypsoralen). Beta-carotene has been used for preventing photosensitivity reactions in patients with porphyrias (metabolic disorders that cause skin eruptions or cause the victim to be particularly sensitive to sunlight). Chloroquine and psoralens have been used for other skin conditions and diseases such as solar urticaria, actinic reticuloid, polymorphous light eruptions, and psoriasis (in conjunction with ultraviolet light therapy).

Although some of the agents occur naturally in food (beta-carotene is found naturally in carrots, oranges, palm oil, and tomatoes) and have been experimentally shown in some cases to provide protection in the range of 400 nm (in excess of UVA), they should not be taken without medical supervision. Products containing canthaxanthin and beta-carotene can be harmful when taken in large doses for long periods of time. In the levels found in the "tanning pills" sold through mail-order houses, they can cause toxic accumulation in the eyes, blood, skin, fatty tissue, and other organs of the body. They may also affect the ability of the eyes to adapt to darkness, and cause long-term damage to the retina. Treatment with or use of any of these agents requires careful prescription of dosage and continuous monitoring by a physician. Used without supervision, they can be deadly.

GUIDELINES FOR SUN SAFETY

The goal of a sun protection program is to stay well under 1 MED of ultraviolet radiation each day. To do this, follow these guidelines:

- Use a sunscreen.
- Wear protective clothing whenever possible, including a wide-brimmed hat, long sleeves, and long pants.
- Avoid sun exposure during the period of most intense sunlight, i.e., 10 am to 3 pm.
- Limit your first seasonal exposure to the sun to only a few minutes, gradually increasing the time by a few minutes on each successive day to allow your skin's melanin reserves sufficient time to come into play.
- At the beach, use an umbrella, sunhat, and protective clothing. Never count on your skin to tell you when to get out of the sun.
- Protect neglected areas, such as the backs of the hands, the tops of the ears, the nape of the neck, bald spots, shoulders, the tip of the nose, feet, and cheeks.
- In the wintertime, you should use a sunscreen because the sun's rays reflect off the snow.
- Be sure to protect your skin on overcast, cool, and breezy days, when you may not feel hot but ultraviolet light is plentiful.
- Use polarized sunglasses, those that screen out up to 400 nm; neutral grays and high contrast browns are the best colors.
- If you are a high-risk individual and/or have an outdoor occupation, use a sunscreen daily.

CHAPTER
9

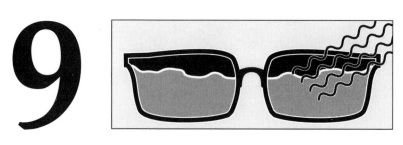

EFFECTIVE EYE PROTECTION: Choosing Sunglasses That Filter Ultraviolet Light

*A*mericans spend almost

one billion dollars a year on sunglasses, usually for comfort and style, often unaware that the glasses they purchase may be harmful to their eyes. Most sunglasses do a fairly good job of reducing glare; however, an estimated 40% of all manufactured sunglasses are inadequate for protecting the eye and surrounding tissues from irradiation by ultraviolet and infrared light. Evidence has been accumulating over the last two decades to show that these forms of radiation are damaging to the eye (Figure 9.1).

SUNLIGHT'S DAMAGING EFFECTS

The damage done to the human lens by ultraviolet rays is a silent, cumulative process causing cataracts and also benign growths, and, rarely, cancerous growths on the conjunctiva (the mucous membrane that covers the inner eyelid and eyeball). Other potential results are malignant eyelid cancers,

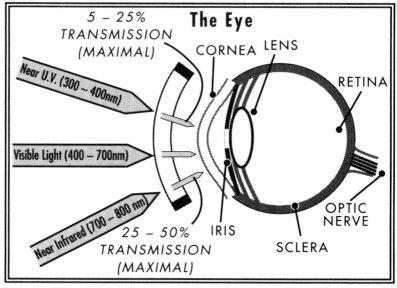

(Figure 9.1)

including malignant melanoma, as well as retinal damage and impaired color perception.

Excessive ultraviolet exposure has been shown to be a significant contributing factor to certain types of skin cancers, including malignant melanomas, all of which can occur on the skin of the eyelids. These cutaneous carcinomas are also more prevalent in individuals with histories of prolonged chronic sun exposure, which reinforces the point that sunlight's effects on the eyes and skin are cumulative—the damage increases over the years.

Damage to the retina has been shown to result from ultraviolet radiation and from light in the blue end of the visible spectrum. The normal human lens protects the retina by absorbing a good portion of ultraviolet radiation (thus increasing the risk of cataract formation, as noted above). Individuals who have lost a lens through cataract extraction have lost a barrier to ultraviolet filtration. Shielding the retina from ultraviolet radiation is particularly important for these people.

RELIABLE STANDARDS

Protective eyewear is as essential for the eyes as a good sunscreen is for the skin. To be effective, sunglasses should absorb the UVA and UVB portions of the spectrum while allowing partial transmission of visible light. Prescription lenses purchased from a reputable optician can incorporate the ultraviolet blocking characteristics if so designated by the prescription. Those who buy over-the-counter glasses have no such assurance. Both The Skin Cancer Foundation and the American National Standards Institute recommend minimum standards of protection. Buyers should look for the inscription "Z-80-3 Standard" or a manufacturer's tag stating that the glasses block ultraviolet radiation. Sunglasses may be either glass or plastic and should be impact-resistant.

The Food and Drug Administration has also developed a system of reliable labels for non-prescription sunglasses. Under this new system, a pair of "cosmetic" sunglasses will block at least 70% of UVB, 20% of UVA, and 60% of visible light, and are suitable for around-town use. "General purpose" glasses block 95% of UVB, 60% of UVA, and 92% of visible light and should be worn for outdoor activities such as hiking, ballgames, or driving. For use in especially bright sunlight, "special purpose" glasses that block 99% of UVB, 60% of UVA, and 97% of visible light are recommended.

The darkest sunglasses are not necessarily good sunglasses. Glasses that are exceptionally dark will cause the pupils to dilate in order to obtain sufficient light, thereby allowing more, not less, ultraviolet radiation into the eye. Neutral grays and high-contrast browns are the most effective tints.

In purchasing sunglasses, fashion will no doubt continue to be an important consideration, but so should the transmission properties of the lenses selected. This should be particularly true for people who have had prolonged, intensive exposure to the sun.

The cost of good protective sunglasses ranges from about $50 to $300 depending on the frame, with an average price of about $85. The payoff in protection of eyesight and surrounding tissues is well worth the price.

10

ON
THE
MARK:
Identifying
Precancerous
Growths

A number of abnormal but relatively harmless skin growths constitute the early warning signs of skin cancer. These may be precancerous lesions, benign tumors that mask or mimic more serious ones, or malignancies as yet confined to the uppermost layers of the skin. They are important to recognize because they give the physician a good headstart in preventing more serious skin cancer. As you become aware of the warning signs, you can participate in your own healthcare through regular self-examinations.

PRECANCEROUS GROWTHS

Skin in a precancerous state is abnormal but not malignant. The term "precancerous" is used because these abnormal areas of skin are much more likely to give rise to malignant growths than is the adjacent normal skin. Precancerous growths are visible to the naked eye, and they look different from normal cells when they are examined under a microscope.

Solar Keratosis

Solar keratosis affects the keratin-filled cells of the skin's stratum corneum, its outer protective layer. It is the result of prolonged exposure to sunlight, usually without adequate protection. Also called actinic—"light-produced"—keratosis, its most frequent victims are fair-complexioned people of middle age or older, with skins that have become coarse, wrinkled, and weatherbeaten as a result of cumulative exposure to the sun.

Although sometimes occurring singly, solar keratoses usually consist of multiple growths. Both single and multiple tumors are slow-growing, tiny (less than 1 cm in diameter), dry, rough, yellowish brown, well-defined scales that do not flake off. They may become thick and horny, and sometimes there are points of bleeding.

Solar keratoses are most frequently found on the backs of the hands, forearms, face, and other areas exposed to the sun. Naked scalps are especially vulnerable — bald-headed persons should wear hats whenever they go out in the sun.

A small percentage of untreated solar keratoses develop into squamous cell carcinoma, so it is essential that these growths be checked periodically and then removed when necessary.

Arsenical Keratosis

Far less common, arsenical keratosis is an accumulation of keratinized tissue that at first resembles numerous small, yellowish corns. These arise most often on the palms, soles, and inner surfaces of the finger and toes and then enlarge and thicken, sometimes increasing in number. Although infrequently seen today, arsenical keratoses usually occur on patients who, though they may not be aware of it, were at some time in their lives exposed to arsenic, either contained in medication or from an industrial or environmental source.

GROWTHS THAT MASK OR MIMIC CANCER

Cutaneous Horns

Small, hard, yellowish-brown growths made up of densely packed keratin tissue are called cutaneous horns (although not all of them actually resemble miniature horns). Like solar keratoses, with which they are sometimes classified, they commonly occur on the exposed parts of the body, particularly the upper part of the face, the ears, and the scalp.

Usually, they occur alone, but multiple cutaneous horns are not rare. Although not malignant in themselves, they must be surgically removed as soon as they are discovered since malignancies have sometimes been found beneath them.

Keratoacanthoma

Keratoacanthoma, a round, rapidly growing tumor, arises mainly on exposed skin areas. The causes of keratoacanthoma are not known, though solar overexposure is still considered the principal one. Keratoacanthoma can also result from burns or cuts on the skin or from repeated contact with tar or mineral oil. Some investigators have suggested that keratoacanthomas may be caused by a virus.

Usually, keratoacanthoma appears as a smooth pimple on

the face or arms, sometimes with a reddish color as the result of distended blood vessels. It grows rapidly, coming to resemble a small golf ball or having the shape of a miniature volcano with a depressed horny or crusted center. It may reach a diameter of 5 cm or more. Usually, it will disappear of its own accord in less than 6 months, leaving a depressed scar.

Although keratoacanthomas are generally benign, they are very difficult to distinguish from malignant squamous cell carcinomas; even under the microscope, they may appear virtually identical. It is therefore strongly recommended that keratoacanthomas be removed without delay, because if misdiagnosed, allowing a squamous cell carcinoma to grow would be detrimental.

EARLY SKIN CANCERS (CARCINOMA IN SITU)

Skin cancers are classified as early cancers, or carcinoma in situ, when malignant changes have occurred but are confined to the epidermis, the top layer of the skin. A biologic barrier called the basement membrane divides the epidermis and dermis and helps to delay deep invasion by malignant cells. It is important that early skin cancers be removed as soon as they are discovered because of their invasive potential.

Bowen's Disease

Bowen's disease, named for the doctor who first classified it, is considered by some experts to be an early stage of squamous cell carcinoma. It is a fairly uncommon type of skin cancer caused either by sunlight or by contact with arsenical compounds.

It can appear on the mucous membranes of the nose and mouth, as well as on the skin, as a slowly enlarging reddish patch with a sharp but irregular outline and areas of crusting within the patches. Its victims are usually middle-aged, although the disease is not uncommon among young adults.

Some researchers believe Bowen's disease to be indicative of internal malignancies. One investigator reported that when the disease arises from contact with arsenic, 15%–25% of those who are afflicted also have internal cancer.

Erythroplasia de Queyrat is a less common variation of Bowen's disease that appears as a red patch on the tip of the penis of uncircumcised men. It may be virus-related. Unlike Bowen's disease, it is not generally indicative of other forms of cancer.

Leukoplakia

Leukoplakia is a disease of the mucous membrane, primarily affecting the mouth and oral cavity. It begins as a benign growth but can develop into squamous cell carcinoma. Leukoplakia appears most frequently on the lips, especially the lower lip, where it resembles a dry, white blotch. In this form the lesion is known as actinic cheilitis and is probably the result of chronic exposure to sunlight.

Another type of leukoplakia appears inside the mouth and on the tongue, sometimes as a tiny spot and sometimes as a large area covering almost the entire oral cavity. It has a smooth, opalescent shimmer, which usually becomes pearly and opaque as it thickens and shrivels but sometimes becomes scaly. This type of leukoplakia has been linked to chronic local irritation that may result from several causes, such as pipe smoking, tobacco chewing, ill-fitting dentures, poor oral hygiene, or even from chewing the lip.

DIAGNOSIS AND BIOPSY

All suspicious areas should be shown to a physician who will observe them under good natural or artificial light. If a site is suspicious for a potential malignancy, a biopsy will be taken. The physician will use 1 of 3 biopsy methods, and the procedure takes only a few minutes at most. The standard method is to take a thin sliver or shave of tissue and place it in a bottle containing formalin, which is then sent to the laboratory for processing. Other methods of obtaining tissue for examination are removal of some tissue with a spoonlike instrument called a curette, or surgically excising a small spectrum of tissue and closing the wound with a suture stitch. If only a small amount of tissue is removed, this method is called incisional biopsy. If the suspected site is small, the physician may elect to do an excisional biopsy in which the total amount of the involved area is removed. Pathology reports are usually available to the patient within 3–7 days. A longer period of time may be required if additional staining in the laboratory is needed to establish a diagnosis.

BASAL CELL CARCINOM
SQUAMOUS CELI

THE MOST COMMON CANCERS: Basal Cell and Squamous Cell Carcinomas

"I had—well, I guess for want of a better word—a pimple on my nose...And it was snipped off...It was indeed a basal cell carcinoma, which is the most common kind...I don't mind telling you all this because I know that medicine has been waging a great campaign to try and convince people to stop broiling themselves in the sun..."

President Ronald Reagan
August 7, 1985

All cancers (also called malignancies or carcinomas) share two qualities. First, their rate of growth is uncontrolled by the normal mechanisms that govern cell reproduction—they tend to grow rapidly. Second, while normal cells tend to "stick together," participating in the formation of their organ, cancerous cells tend to disperse; isolated cells make their way into the bloodstream or lymphatic system and are carried to other parts of the body where they lodge and continue to reproduce rapidly. This spreading process, called metastasis, is extremely dangerous. Cancer causes disease either by displacing other cells and disturbing their functions or by competing with them for nutrients.

Virtually every cancer begins with an alteration (called a mutation) in the genetic material of a single cell. All later generations of that cell are cancerous, too. Mutations may occur because of exposure to radiation (the sun, x-rays), certain chemicals (those in cigarette smoke or asbestos), or even viruses. In the case of most skin cancer, the sun is the chief cancer-causing agent.

There are three major types of skin cancer. Two of these, basal cell carcinoma and squamous cell carcinoma, are the most common of all cancers. Although they seldom metastasize, they are malignant, and both types will continue to grow if not destroyed or surgically removed. They can cause the loss of an eye, ear, nose, or large portions of the face or body parts if not diagnosed and treated early.

The third type, malignant melanoma, occurs less frequently. It is much more dangerous, though, because it grows quickly and is more likely to metastasize to other organs of the body, thus becoming life-threatening. However, because malignant melanoma is visible on the skin, it is one of the easiest tumors to find and one of the simplest to cure, if it found and removed early.

BASAL CELL CARCINOMA

Basal cell carcinoma (also known as basal cell epithelioma) is the most common type of skin cancer. As its name indicates, it originates in the basal cells of the epidermis. This tumor most often appears on the face. Although the growth does interfere to some extent with normal development of the skin, it is the slowest spreading of all tumors. It rarely metastasizes, and fortunately has a high cure rate. Learn to recognize the warning signs of basal cell carcinoma. These are listed below, and also illustrated in color photographs 1 through 6.

• A skin growth that increases in size and appears pearly and translucent, often with a rolled edge and a dent in the middle.

• A spot or patch that continues to itch, hurt, crust, scab, or bleed.

• An open sore or wound that does not heal or persists for more than 4 weeks, or closes and then reopens.

A few investigators have gone so far as to say that basal cell carcinoma is not "bad" cancer, but medical evidence has disproven this statement. Not infrequently, basal cell carcinoma can be quite aggressive—5%–10% resist the initial attempt at removal, and further efforts to eradicate the tumor can cause disfigurement and the loss of vital organs.

The incidence of basal cell carcinoma increases with age, although this cancer can attack any age group. Following the general pattern of skin cancer incidence, it appears with greatest frequency among fair-skinned people. Scientists believe that its primary cause is exposure to sunlight, though other factors still unknown may be involved. Basal cell carcinomas are classified clinically according to characteristic features and colors.

Nodular or Noduloulcerative

Nodular basal cell carcinoma is the most common type. The tumor usually resembles a smooth, round, waxy pimple, pale yellow or pearl gray, and may vary in size from a few millimeters to 1 centimeter (slightly more than one-third of an inch). The blood vessels inside the nodule may be chronically dilated, a condition called telangiectasia, and the skin covering the nodule is often stretched so thin that the slightest injury will cause it to bleed. Often the tumor appears depressed in the middle and shows ulceration. It is called a rodent ulcer. As the tumor grows, it destroys structures in its path, including nerves and blood vessels. Large tumors are quite distinctive and easily diagnosed, but smaller ones are more difficult to differentiate from benign skin conditions. Often, these smaller tumors are misdiagnosed as warts, moles, psoriasis, or fever sores.

Pigmented

Pigmented basal cell carcinoma is similar to nodular basal cell carcinoma, but is more likely to appear in people with dark hair and dark eyes. As its name implies, the tumor cells of this growth are almost black and can easily be mistaken for the more aggressive malignant melanoma.

Fibrosing

Fibrosing basal cell carcinoma is also referred to as morphea-like carcinoma. This tumor sometimes looks like the nonmalignant skin condition called scleroderma, in which the skin becomes shiny, thickened, and rigid. A fairly uncommon type of skin cancer, it can be difficult to eradicate because of invisible, rootlike extensions of the tumorous cells into underlying tissue.

This fibrosing type of tumor begins as a flat or slightly depressed, shiny, hard, yellow-white patch with an irregular border. It seldom crusts or ulcerates. Sometimes, it may be present for many years without noticeably growing or being recognized by either patient or physician. However, more commonly the lesion grows fairly rapidly, reaching a diameter of several centimeters within a few months.

Fibroepithelioma

Fibroepithelioma is a rare type of basal cell carcinoma appearing as one or more slightly elevated, reddish lesions that resemble skin tags. Usually they appear on the back.

Superficial

Superficial basal cell carcinoma is the least common type. It is a progressively spreading, slow-growing cancer that differs greatly from other types of this disease. Without confirmation of its diagnosis by biopsy (microscopic examination of cells), it is often mistaken for other skin conditions, including fungus, eczema, or psoriasis.

The skin cancer tumors are red, with a slightly raised, sometimes ulcerated or crusted surface, often bordered with pearly, threadlike formations. Larger and older tumors may thicken, developing into a nodular type of basal cell carcinoma.

Tumors appear most frequently as patches on the torso. When they develop on the face and neck, they tend to be extensive.

BASAL CELL NEVUS SYNDROME

This condition, commonly referred to as nevoid basal cell carcinoma syndrome, is relatively rare and often occurs in persons with a family history of the disease. Unlike other skin cancer conditions, this syndrome may develop during childhood or adolescence, and as many as 50–100 cancers may be involved. Sometimes the skin cancers increase in number as the individual reaches adulthood. Clinically, they have the same appearance as other basal cell carcinomas.

SQUAMOUS CELL CARCINOMA

Squamous cell carcinomas occur less frequently than basal cell carcinomas, commonly appearing in areas of skin damaged by either the sun or by some other condition. Rarely does squamous cell carcinoma arise spontaneously on what appears to be normal skin. The tumors originate from squamous cells of the epidermis and usually remain confined to the upper level of the skin.

Compared to basal cell carcinoma, squamous cell carcinoma grows faster and is more likely to metastasize. In the small percentage of cases where it spreads to other parts of the body, it is frequently fatal. This possibility makes early diagnosis vital, but fortunately squamous cell carcinoma is often preceded by solar keratosis, an easily identified precancerous lesion.

When it is of solar origin, squamous cell carcinoma usually appears on skin that already shows damage in the form of wrinkling, pigmentation, loss of elasticity, and frequently, solar keratoses. Squamous cell tumors also appear on burn and scar sites, and areas of chronic inflammatory skin conditions (where they may go unnoticed) as well as on radiation-damaged skin. Contact with tars, petroleum distillates, or arsenic is another possible cause of the cancer. Some investigators believe that the tendency to develop squamous cell carcinoma may have an hereditary component.

Squamous cell tumors are thick, rough, horny, and shallow when they develop. Occasionally they will ulcerate, with a raised border and a crusted surface over a raised, pebbly, granular base. Among Caucasians, squamous cell carcinomas are most prevalent on areas that have received heavy exposure to the sun, such as the hands, forearms, and forehead, with the lower lip and outer part of the ear especially vulnerable. (See color photographs 7 through 11 for examples of squamous cell carcinoma.) Squamous cell carcinoma in darker-skinned individuals frequently develops due to some preexisting chronic skin lesion.

Any bump or open sore in areas of chronic inflammatory skin lesions indicates the possibility of squamous cell carcinoma and mandates an immediate visit to a physician.

BASOSQUAMOUS CELL CARCINOMA

Squamous and basal cell carcinomas can coexist as one tumor growth at the same time. Clinically it will appear as a basal cell or squamous cell carcinoma. Difficulty with diagnosis may be compounded when a tumor reveals both types of cells under the microscope. Therefore, a category called basosquamous cell carcinoma was established. Most dermatopathologists (physicians who specialize in the microscopic structure of tissue) state that a true combined or transitional form is unlikely to exist. Basosquamous cell carcinomas are believed by some researchers to have a greater tendency to metastasize. These tumors have to be treated immediately and aggressively.

SKIN CANCER IN BLACKS

Squamous cell carcinoma represents more than two-thirds of all skin cancers in blacks. It afflicts more black men than black women—almost a 2:1 ratio—and appears most frequently on the face and neck. It may occur in the site of an existing scar or keloid, burn, or other lesion. Other predisposing factors may be lupus or osteomyelitis. Blacks with chronic inflammatory conditions or scarring dermatoses or other poorly healing lesions such as an ulcer are also at risk, as are black albinos.

Basal cell carcinoma is uncommon in blacks, but does occur on sun-exposed skin. As with squamous cell carcinoma, predisposing factors such as concomitant disease add to the risk of developing this cancer. Two-thirds of basal cell carcinoma in blacks occurs in the head and neck region, but it can also occur in the anus, prepuce, and nipple areas. There is an equal ratio of occurrence in men and women.

Because both basal and squamous cell carcinoma are particularly aggressive in blacks, any translucent, pigmented pimple-like lesions warrant prompt medical attention.

CHAPTER

12

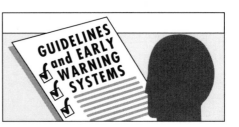

MALIGNANT MELANOMA:
Guidelines
and
Early
Warning
Systems

BASAL CELL CARCINOMA

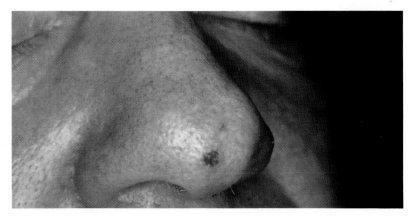

1. Basal cell carcinoma: Look for an open sore that bleeds, oozes, or crusts and remains open for three or more weeks, or heals and recurs.

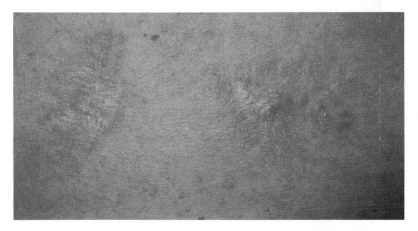

2. Also look for a reddish patch or irritated area. The patch may crust, itch, or hurt, or it may persist with no noticeable discomfort.

BASAL CELL CARCINOMA

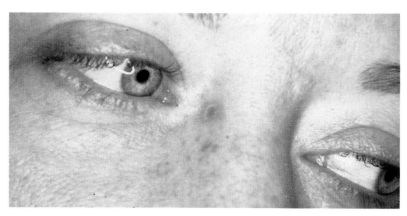

3. A smooth growth like this one should be checked by your physician.

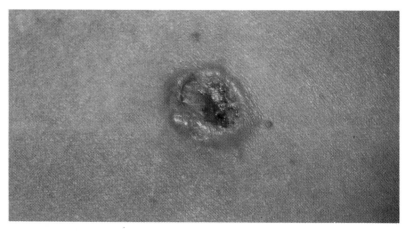

4. Another danger sign is a growth with an elevated, rolled border and an indentation in the center. As the growth slowly enlarges, tiny blood vessels may develop on the surface.

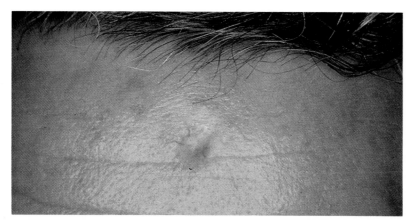

5. A thready scar-like area that often has poorly defined borders; although a less frequent sign of basal cell carcinoma, this can indicate the presence of an aggressive tumor.

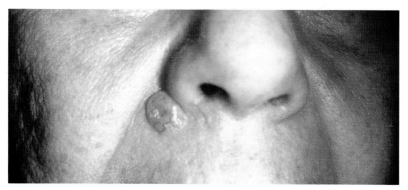

6. A shiny bump, or nodule, that is pearly or translucent and is often pink, red, or white, is a warning sign.

SQUAMOUS CELL CARCINOMA

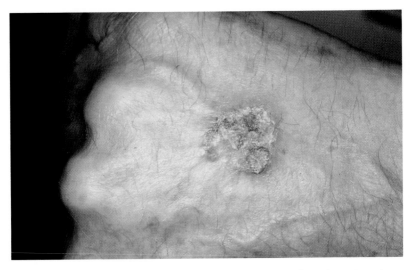

7. Squamous cell carcinoma: Look for a persistent, scaly red patch with irregular borders that sometimes crusts or bleeds.

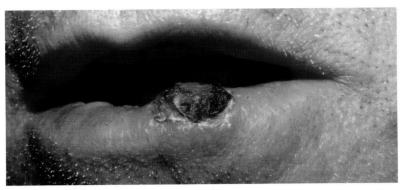

8. It may also appear as an elevated growth with a central depression that occasionally bleeds.

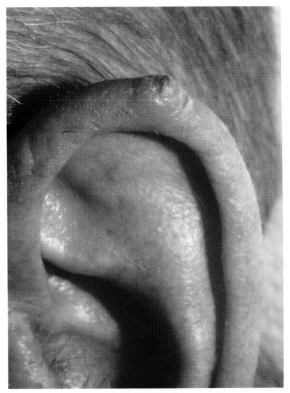

9. Some squamous cell tumors are wart-like. They crust and occasionally bleed.

SQUAMOUS CELL CARCINOMA

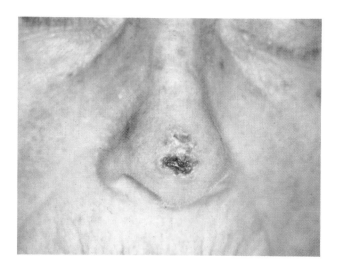

10/11. Open sores like these that bleed and crust and persist for weeks may be squamous cell carcinoma.

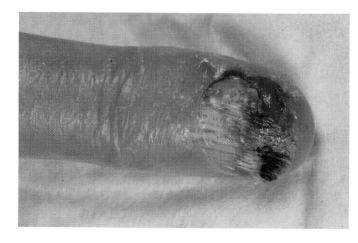

MALIGNANT MELANOMA

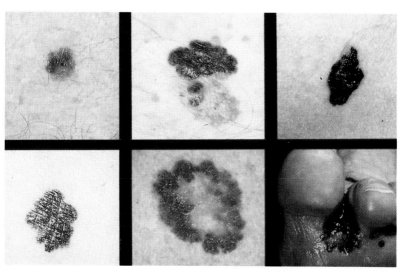

12. Six examples of malignant melanoma. Common characteristics are asymmetry, irregular borders, various colors within the same growth, and diameter larger than ¼ inch.

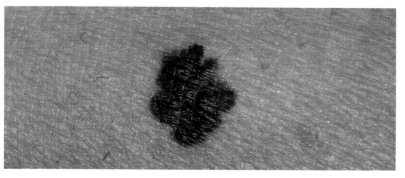

13. Malignant melanoma in its early stage, when it can be easily treated. Many melanomas arise in pre-existing moles, but not all.

MALIGNANT MELANOMA

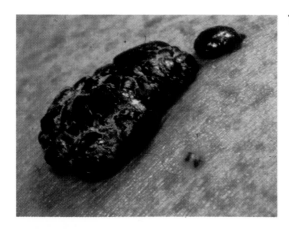

14. Advanced melanoma: At this point treatment is not always successful; the disease may quickly spread to other parts of the body, in which case it is often fatal.

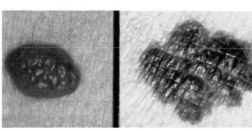

15. A single word, "change," should alert us to the possibility of malignant melanoma. Left, a normal mole; right, malignant melanoma

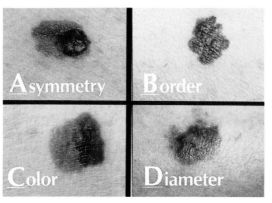

16. As you examine your moles and spots, The Skin Cancer Foundation suggests you remember the ABCD's of moles and melanomas.

Medical records from the time of Hippocrates, Father of Medicine, describe the "black tumors" we know as malignant melanoma, the potentially lethal form of skin cancer that results from an uncontrolled growth of melanocytes, the pigment-producing cells in the bottom layer of the epidermis. Although progress has been made in diagnosis and treatment of this disease, we still know far too little about its causes.

INCIDENCE

Malignant melanoma comprises only 5% of all skin cancers, yet its annual incidence—the number of new cases diagnosed—has increased almost 1200% since the 1930s and is increasing at a faster rate than any other cancer in the United States. It is currently estimated that by the year 2000, one in 90 Americans will develop malignant melanoma during his or her lifetime (Figure 12.1). This year approximately 27,600 people in this country will develop the disease, and 6,300 will die.

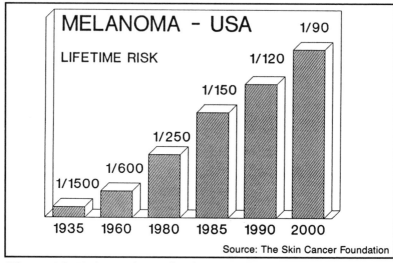

(Figure 12.1) The incidence of malignant melanoma has increased almost 1200% since the 1930s.

Malignant melanoma strikes earlier than other skin cancers, sometimes even before age 30. It affects men and women equally, although women have a better survival rate before menopause, perhaps due to the protection afforded them by estrogen levels. Whites have a 10 times greater risk than blacks of developing melanoma, and their overall lifetime risk increased by 50% between 1950 and 1980.

Despite these staggering figures, malignant melanomas are being diagnosed earlier and treated more successfully: 50 years ago, three of five persons diagnosed with malignant melanoma died within 5 years. Today four of five survive more than 5 years. However, much remains to be done, especially in teaching people to recognize the warning signs of the disease and to seek prompt medical attention when changes are noted in a mole, or when a new mole appears in adulthood. (See color photographs 12 through 14.)

CAUSES OF MALIGNANT MELANOMA

What causes malignant melanoma? As yet, science does not know the answer with certainty, but a number of factors appear to be linked with the disease: solar overexposure, the presence of many moles (especially unusual ones or those present at birth), genetic predisposition, previous malignancy, chemical carcinogens, etc. The list is long and probably a combination of factors will prove responsible.

Beyond these general considerations, several specific factors identify individuals who are prone to develop this tumor. People at high risk are those who have:

- a family history of malignant melanoma
- a previous melanoma
- many moles
- unusual—"dysplastic"—moles (often larger than one-third inch, irregular in shape, and multi-colored)
- fair skin, light hair, and light eye color, and a tendency to sunburn easily and to tan with difficulty
- very large brown moles at birth
- a record of painful or blistering sunburns, especially when young
- indoor occupations and outdoor recreational habits
- considerable outdoor exposure, especially while living in sunny regions

The Sun

Solar radiation clearly plays a role in malignant melanoma, although its extent is not fully defined. Like other skin cancers, malignant melanomas are linked to factors that influence sun exposure, including nearness to the equator, high altitude, low humidity, and frequency of sunny, cloudless days.

Sunlight probably causes melanoma through its mutagenic effect as well as a possible role in suppressing the immune system.

Most malignant melanomas appear on the back and legs. They occur 3 times as frequently on the legs of women and 6 times as frequently on the ears of men, obviously reflecting patterns of dress and hairstyle that affect sun exposure. Malignant melanoma can appear elsewhere—often on the trunk, at times in the eye, on the palms, and on the soles especially in blacks.

The incidence of malignant melanoma is dramatically escalated in areas where light-skinned persons are exposed to large amounts of solar radiation. Overall, in the United States the incidence of malignant melanoma in whites is 12 in 100,000, but in Queensland, Australia, an area of intense sun inhabited by fair-skinned people whose parents or grandparents migrated from the United Kingdom, the incidence is 44 in 100,000, nearly 4 times as high! Inhabitants of Western Australia who spent their early childhood there have an incidence greater than those who immigrated at a later age, underscoring the cumulative nature of sun damage, and the fact that much damage is done during childhood.

Recent studies show that the risk of malignant melanoma is doubled in persons who have one or more blistering sunburns in childhood, as it is in people with type I skin.

Not all research studies are so clear-cut. Indoor workers and persons in higher socioeconomic brackets have incidences of malignant melanoma that are higher than those of outdoor workers. It is probable that the incidence of malignant melanoma in office workers is due to the intense, brief bursts of sunlight they experience in leisure hours.

A minority of researchers believes that the sun is of

minimal importance in inducing malignant melanoma or that it acts chiefly as a trigger in lesions with preexisting malignant potential. Most, however, believe, as I do, that solar radiation is a direct cause of at least some, if not many, malignant melanomas.

Nevi (Moles)

Moles are common growths containing cells related to pigment-producing melanocytes. About 75%–80% of whites have one or more moles. Some have hundreds. Moles have no known function, and it is not known why they form. They initially appear in the first year of life and continue to appear until age 40; many then begin to disappear.

Usually moles are flat and round, with a regular border. They may be slightly elevated, and may range in color from pink to slightly darker than surrounding skin to dark brown and black. Most moles are benign and show no change during a lifetime. It is seldom necessary to remove them unless they are constantly irritated by clothing or are large and cosmetically unacceptable.

Because 20% of malignant melanomas begin in moles, and because early melanoma may be almost indistinguishable from ordinary brown or black moles, any new pigmented growth or a change in an existing growth is suspect no matter what its appearance.

Dysplastic Nevi

Dysplastic nevi are moles that are atypical. These unusual moles are either flat or somewhat elevated. Their pigment is invariably variegated and uneven. Their borders are often irregular. Frequently they are larger than 6 mm (one-quarter inch), that is, larger than the size of a pencil eraser.

It has been reported that approximately 5%–7% of Americans have dysplastic nevi, usually appearing by age 10. If none are apparent by age 20, their development is unlikely. Their cause is unclear, although a genetic component exists: family members of people with dysplastic nevi are 8–10 times more likely to develop them. They may also occur, however, in persons with no family history of dysplastic nevi.

Because of their potential for malignant change, dysplastic nevi should be carefully monitored by a physician. Not all change is malignant, however. For suspicious lesions, total removal is recommended. This eliminates the risk of melanoma in that particular mole. If no suspicion of malignancy exists, dysplastic nevi need not be removed except for cosmetic reasons. Because persons with dysplastic nevi may also have intraocular nevi, regularly scheduled eye examinations are strongly recommended.

The dyplastic nevus syndrome is still under investigation and will undergo further development as our knowledge about these moles increases. However, since dyplastic nevi identify a portion of the population more prone to develop malignant melanoma than people who do not have these moles, it is prudent to follow them carefully and to undergo regular medical examinations by a physician specializing in skin diseases.

Congenital Moles

Congenital nevi occur in about 1%–2% of infants. Readily apparent at birth, they range in color from red to brown to black, and may cover a small area or up to one-third or more of the infant's skin. Some congenital moles become malignant. If they are small and smooth and lightly pigmented (and therefore more easily followed), they should be regularly checked and evaluated by your dermatologist.

Giant congenital nevi are cause for concern. Malignant melanoma will probably develop in 5%–10% of these, so surgery should be performed in infancy. Any infant with a congenital nevus should be followed from birth onward. No matter what the size of the nevus, any change, especially lumpiness or darkening, should be considered grounds for surgery. Follow-up should continue after surgery as well.

Genetic Factors

Genetic factors probably play a greater role in the development of melanoma than in any other skin malignancies. Studies have shown that as many as 1 in 20 (or more) cases of malignant melanoma are genetic in origin. For this reason, the grandparents, parents, aunts/uncles, siblings, and children of melanoma patients should also be examined.

Other Factors

Other factors that have been considered to play a role in causing melanoma are: oncogenic (cancer-causing) viruses; industrial or environmental pollutants; chemical carcinogens, hormones; and even fluorescent lights. Further research should be aimed at sorting out and explaining the individual and combined causal roles of all these factors in malignant melanoma and in other skin cancers.

THICKNESS OF MELANOMA

Malignant melanomas are catagorized by their thickness. With the aid of a microscope, the thickness of the lesion is measured from an upper layer of the epidermis (the stratum granulosum) to the deepest point of its penetration into the skin. This dimension is the best prognosticator of the type and extent of surgery needed to ensure removal of the entire growth, the amount of safety margin required, and the need for removal of regional lymph nodes.

"Thin" melanomas are defined as those that penetrate less than 0.75 mm. If malignant melanoma is removed at this stage, cure is virtually certain because cancerous change is limited to the lesion itself. "Intermediate" thickness, 0.76 to 3 mm, poses a greater risk. However, overall prognosis for cure for this category of melanomas is still somewhat good (85% overall). In "thick" melanomas (i.e. thicker than 3 mm) the risk of local recurrence and for distant metastasis to other body organs is substantially greater (overall 60% or greater).

Currently, approximately 50% of all malignant melanomas are of the low-risk type. If a biopsy reveals malignant melanoma, removal of all cells of the lesion is mandatory to prevent metastasis to the surrounding tissue or to internal organs such as lungs, liver, or brain. In thick lesions, however, even wide and deep local removal does not guarantee that malignant melanoma will not recur or develop in another area.

TYPES OF MALIGNANT MELANOMA

Melanomas have generally been classified into two main groups: those that invade deeply from the very beginning (nodular) and those that spread superficially for some time before they invade deeply.

Nodular Melanoma

Of all melanomas, 10%–15% are nodular in type and invade deeply from the very beginning. Nodular melanoma usually occurs between the ages of 30 and 60 and may appear anywhere on the body. These melanomas form nodules, dome-shaped bumps that vary in color from dark brown to red, blue, or black. Sometimes the nodule is skin colored or only slightly tinged with brown color. The texture may be shiny, scaly, or fissured. This type of melanoma is the most aggressive and has the poorest prognosis because, on average, it is a thicker tumor.

Horizontally Spreading Malignant Melanomas

There are three basic types of melanomas that spread mostly horizontally before they invade very deeply: superficial spreading melanoma, lentigo maligna melanoma, and acral-lentiginous melanoma.

Superficial spreading melanoma usually develops between the ages of 45 and 60 on sun-exposed skin. It is often in the shape of a maple leaf, with a patchwork pigmentation of black, gray, pink, red, tan, blue, or white. These melanomas usually occur on the upper back in both sexes and on the legs in women. They may often spread superficially for years before a papule or nodule develops within the patch or plaque. Once a nodule develops, superficial spreading malignant melanoma behaves like nodular malignant melanoma, thickness for thickness.

Lentigo maligna melanoma, or melanotic freckle, is a less common type of horizontally spreading malignant melanoma that may begin at any age but commonly appears in the elderly as a light brown facial lesion. Because a nodule tends to develop quite late in lentigo maligna melanoma, it is slightly less threatening for some time than a nodular malignant melanoma, which tends to grow more rapidly. However, once a nodule develops, prognosis is equally poor, thickness for thickness.

Acral-lentiginous melanoma, which accounts for only 3% of all malignant melanomas, appears exclusively on the palms, fingers, soles, and toes (including the skin sites under the nails). A greater percentage of melanomas occur in blacks and Asians in these acral areas as compared with whites.

Like all horizontally spreading malignant melanoma, acral-lentiginous melanoma may spread superficially for months and even years, often undetected or ignored owing to its location. It frequently has some of the characteristics of lentigo maligna melanoma.

Other Melanomas

Familial malignant melanoma is characterized by early onset, a high frequency of multiple primary melanomas, a greater likelihood of malignancies other than skin, and yet a higher survival rate than that of nonfamilial melanomas.

Melanomas may arise on mucous membranes and also in the back of the eye. In blacks the proportion of melanomas on mucous membranes is greater than in whites. These often go unnoticed for long periods of time because of the location. They are frequently lethal.

As you can see, melanomas take many forms. Because growths and lesions of all kinds so frequently resemble each other, the only positive way to identify and therefore effectively treat any form of skin cancer is with a biopsy. Once the condition is accurately identified, proper treatment can be pursued.

PROTECTING YOURSELF FROM MALIGNANT MELANOMA

My patients give various reasons for their delay in seeking advice about a suspect lesion. Some are unaware of it—it may be on their back or hidden by hair. Others underestimate its significance, believing that a slight change in a lesion is of no great consequence. Some procrastinate because they are busy, they deny its importance, or they are afraid (denial).

If you have any mole or other pigmented lesion that undergoes change of any kind, your worst enemy is delay. (See color photograph 15.) Your best chance of successful treatment and cure is an immediate visit to your physician. Use the following guidelines to help you identify malignant melanoma on your skin.

ABCD's of Malignant Melanoma

The Skin Cancer Foundation recommends learning the ABCD's of malignant melanoma. (See color photograph 16.) In any mole or pigmented lesion, watch for the following:

•**A**symmetry

•**B**order irregularity

•**C**olor variegation (brown, black, blue, red, white)

•**D**iameter enlargement - diameter over one-quarter inch

In addition, new pigmentation in skin surrounding a "mole" is suspect, as are new pigmented moles or areas in previously normal skin.

Warning Signs

Any one or more of the following changes occurring in a new or existing pigmented (tan, brown) area of the skin, or in a mole, may indicate the presence of a malignant melanoma:

- **Change in size:** especially sudden or continuous enlargement.
- **Change in color:** especially multiple shades of tan, brown, dark brown, black; the mixing of red, white, and blue; or the spreading of color from the edge into the surrounding skin.
- **Change in shape:** developing an irregular, notched border, which used to be regular.
- **Change in elevation:** the raising of a part of a pigmented area that used to be flat or only slightly elevated.
- **Change in surrounding skin:** redness, swelling, or the developing of colored blemishes next to the pigmented area.
- **Change in surface:** scaliness, erosion, oozing, crusting, ulceration, or bleeding.
- **Change in sensation:** itchiness, tenderness, or pain.
- **Change in consistency:** softening or hardening.

Know Your Skin

You can best avoid the potentially lethal effects of malignant melanoma by knowing the normal condition of your skin and examining it regularly once every few months for any new growth or change in existing growths. All of us should have regular yearly physical examinations, including an examination of the skin by a doctor.

Changes in Hormone Balance

Sometimes, patients with dysplastic moles go through periods in which their moles are changing quickly and many new moles are appearing, such as in adolescence and pregnancy. During such episodes of "increased mole activity," moles should be watched with special care and doctor visits increased to every 3 months.

Extra doctor checkups may also be required during adolescence and pregnancy. The use of drugs, such as oral contraceptives or estrogens for treatment of menopausal symptoms, should be avoided by higher risk individuals, if possible. Although the evidence on which this suggestion is based is not very strong, it is enough to make concern worthwhile.

Early Warning System

It is now possible to accurately predict which malignant melanomas are curable and which are not. Malignant melanomas that are removed at an early stage, when they are less than three-quarters of a millimeter thick (about 1/32nd of an inch), are cured in virtually all cases. However, thicker melanomas have less favorable prognoses.

You should examine your skin regularly, as often as once a month if you have had a previous skin cancer or have any of the risk factors aforementioned. Chapter 20 will guide you in performing a total body skin examination. Watch for changes in size, shape, or color, for a sore that does not heal or for a patch that crusts, oozes, or bleeds.

Recommendations for High-Risk Patients

Persons having any of the following factors are at high risk for malignant melanoma and should examine their skin monthly:

- Moles (changing, present from birth, unusual, large number)
- Type I skin (burn easily; unable to tan)
- Family and/or personal history of malignant melanoma
- Blistering sunburn(s) in childhood or teens

Yearly monitoring by a physician of congenital moles, dysplastic nevi, or anyone with a family or personal history of malignant melanoma is the wisest course.

For diagnosis of suspect lesions, the physician may elect to do a biopsy, a minor surgical procedure that will provide results within a week. If malignancy exists, proper treatment can then be started immediately.

13

WHO GETS SKIN CANCER: The Differences Between Men and Women

During the past 24 years that I have been practicing skin cancer surgery at New York University Medical Center, I have discovered some interesting things about my patients and about the proportion of skin cancer in men versus women.

From 1965 to 1987 we collected information on 16,620 skin cancers we treated by Mohs micrographic surgery. Analysis of the data we acquired confirmed many of my assumptions about this disease and has proven to be a useful resource in determining who gets skin cancer and at what ages, the types and locations of lesions in men as compared with women, and the chances for cure.

Some of our findings were compared with the National Cancer Institute (NCI) Report of 1983, prepared by Joseph Scotto, Thomas R. Fears, and Joseph F. Fraumeni, Jr., which presents statistics on 31,578 cases of non-melanoma skin cancers collected from eight regional centers in the United States.

SKIN CANCERS MORE COMMON IN MEN

The number of men with skin cancers in our practice slightly outnumbered women 8,826 to 7,777; that is, 53.2% were men and 46.8% were women. Our figures vary very little from those of the NCI report, which also reveals a slightly higher prevalence for men. This may reflect an occupational hazard, as men are more likely to work outdoors (see graph).

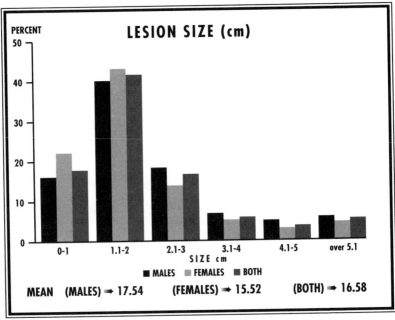

(Figure 13.1)

AGE: ALMOST TWICE AS MANY IN YOUNGER WOMEN

Even though skin cancer is more common in men, we treated more women in the under-40 age group. Percentage-wise, almost twice as many were women: 7% women versus 4.4% men were under the age of 40. The average age for men was 61.5 years, and for women it was 60.7 years. There were three patients treated who were over the age of 95 (two women and one man, aged 97 years).

EARLIER DETECTION

When patients were referred for Mohs surgery prior to 1980, only 12.6% of the lesions treated were less than one centimeter (approximately one-half inch) in diameter. Today, 20% of the lesions we treat are that size and almost 50% of all lesions treated are less than 2 cm. Obviously, patients, or their physicians, are recognizing skin cancers earlier and are seeking treatment for them earlier, while they are still relatively small in size. The mean size for women is 1.5 cm and for men 1.7 cm. Why we see more women than men with smaller lesions is not known. Women may become aware of a growth on the face sooner than men do, and possibly seek medical attention more promptly (see graph).

LESION DURATION

In our 1980 study, which evaluated 15 years of Mohs surgery cases, 26.7% of patients reported that the lesion had existed for less than a year. In our more recent study, completed in 1987, a much larger percentage (63.6%) of patients said they had had the lesion for less than a year. More men than women gave a history of having the lesion for less than one year. We know that lesions in men are usually larger (1.7 cm for men, 1.5 cm for women). Again, it may be that men are less likely to notice the presence of a growth on the skin, or, if they do, they may be more likely to deny its existence or gravity.

SITES OF THE BODY

In our study and in those of other researchers, men developed basal cell carcinomas on the scalp and ears more often than women. Undoubtedly this reflects the difference in the amount of hair and the hairstyles of the sexes. Lesions around the eyes, which comprise about 20% of all skin cancers, occur with equal frequency in both sexes. Women, however, have a much higher percentage of lesions on the neck and lips than men do. One might assume that cosmetics would be effective in blocking out skin cancers from these areas, but until recently few cosmetics or lipsticks contained sunscreens.

Basal cell carcinomas occur more frequently on the trunk and upper extremities in men and on the lower extremities in women, again reflecting the varying patterns of dress; more men than women are apt to bare the upper torso fully, and women far more frequently are bare-legged.

Men have more squamous cell carcinomas on the scalp, ears, and arms, again reflecting patterns of dress and hairstyle. Yet, men also have more squamous cell carcinomas on the legs. Women have more squamous cell carcinomas on the nose: 60% for women versus 40% for men. The reasons for these differences are unclear.

TYPES OF SUN EXPOSURE A FACTOR

In our 1980 study, we learned that our male patients had more basal cell carcinomas on the left side of the face and that the women had more on the right side of the face. We postulated that men were more often the drivers of automobiles and women more often the passengers. Our more recent study, however, shows that the incidences of basal cell carcinomas are greater on the left side of the face in both sexes. Can we assume that women are now in the driver's seat as often as men are?

At the same time, we compared the areas of the body most often protected from the sun in both sexes: the trunk and the chest. In men, there was an increase in the number of lesions on the left side of the body; in women, the frequency was equally divided between the right and the left sides.

Size and Location Affect Cure

Our general cure rate using Mohs surgery is 97.4%. Size and location are the most important factors in cure rates. The smaller the lesion, the greater the chance of cure. With lesions less than 1 cm (approximately one-half inch) our cure rate was approximately 99.6%. With lesions greater than 5 cm the cure rate was 92%. The ears and the retroauricular area are the most difficult sites in which to eradicate skin cancers. In the retroauricular area (the area behind the ear extending to the ear lobe) we had a recurrence rate of 14%. The recurrence rate in the ears was 4.8%. The higher occurrence rate in ears and retroauricular areas may have its origin in their embryological development. In such areas containing many different fusion planes and layers, the tumor may penetrate more readily to deeper levels. In the ears, the tumors did not penetrate the cartilage but can extend a considerable distance away from their initial site.

The consideration of gender as reflected in cure rate was clearly related to the larger lesions found in male patients. If the lesions had been treated earlier, cure rates would have been higher. However, the younger the patient, the more difficult the cancer was to eradicate. Tumors in younger patients may be more aggressive. Further study may provide some answers.

EDUCATION RESULTS IN HIGHER CURE RATES

It is encouraging to conclude that patients are seeking treatment earlier, usually in less than a year; and that they are now first seen with smaller lesions, more than one-half of them less than 1 inch in diameter. Clearly, educational programs such as those conducted by The Skin Cancer Foundation are effective in promoting early diagnosis and treatment. The fortunate result is that we are now able to achieve an even higher cure rate in treating skin cancers of the face and body.

CHAPTER

14

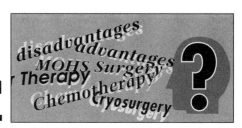

SKIN CANCER TREATMENT: What Are the Options?

*T*here is no one best method to treat all skin cancers and precancerous conditions. The choice of therapy is determined by the location, type, and size of the lesion, and whether it is a primary tumor or a recurrent one. Other considerations are the age, health, and preference of the patient. Finally, the physician's familiarity with the technique is also important.

For a tumor on the body, one might choose a treatment that has a high cure rate and is painless but that may leave a conspicuous scar. However, for the face, the same individual might insist on a treatment that leaves the least possible scar even though that treatment is painful and carries greater risk of a recurrence.

Almost all treatment can be performed in the physician's office or in special outpatient surgical facilities. Most skin cancer removal can be done using a local anesthetic, although larger tumors sometimes require general anesthesia and hospital admission.

Current methods of treating skin cancer are:

- Excisional surgery (excising or cutting out the tumor)
- Irradiation (using x-rays to destroy the tumor)
- Curettage (scraping out the cancerous tissue)
- Electrosurgery (tissue removal with an electric needle)
- Curettage-electrodesiccation (combining the above two methods)
- Cryosurgery (freezing the tumor)
- Chemotherapy, either topical or systemic (chemical treatment either directly on the tumor or internally by pill or injection)
- Laser therapy (removal with laser light)
- Mohs micrographic surgery

Cure rates for most of the modes of therapy are excellent—approaching 85%–95% for primary basal cell carcinomas.

Curettage-electrodesiccation and excisional surgery are the most widely used, although radiation is often employed in elderly persons who cannot or will not tolerate surgery. Use of newer techniques such as cryosurgery and chemotherapy is growing as these treatments demonstrate their effectiveness. Laser therapy, now used only experimentally, has shown promising results. Systemic chemotherapy is primarily used in conjunction with surgery for metastatic malignant melanomas.

Mohs micrographic surgery is an effective, well-established method for treating difficult and recurring skin cancers. Although it is not widely available, it offers excellent cosmetic results and a higher cure rate than any of the other types of treatment. In Mohs micrographic surgery, the tumor is removed with the guidance of a microscope, resulting in removal of the malignancy with minimal loss of normal tissue. Chapter 16 discusses Mohs surgery in detail.

EXCISIONAL SURGERY

Surgical excision is widely used to treat all types of skin cancer. It is the treatment of choice for malignant melanoma.

At its best—given an experienced surgeon and a small, well-placed tumor—surgery can offer results that are often both medically and cosmetically excellent. However, the technique requires considerable skill; the physician must be something of an artist to plan the excision in such a way as to hide the scars as much as possible in the folds and creases of the skin. Such planning is particularly important for tumors on the face. It is easier to conceal the scars in the lines and wrinkles of older patients than in the smoother skin of young people.

Technique

The physician begins by outlining the tumor with a marking pen. A "safety margin" of healthy-looking tissue will be included, because it is not possible to determine with the naked eye how far microscopic strands of tumor may extend beyond the visible edge. Then the intended line of incision is drawn; this is usually about 3 times as long as it is wide so that the skin can be sewn together again after surgery. Marking is usually done before the area is anesthetized, since swelling from the anesthetic causes distortion.

After the lines are drawn, the physician injects a local anesthetic, waits about 10 minutes, then cuts along the lines he has drawn. He puts the tissue removed into a specimen bottle and closes the wound. The entire procedure takes only about 30 minutes for smaller lesions.

Closing and suturing the wound requires a high degree of skill, which can make all the difference between a scar that is barely noticeable and one that is disfiguring. Many patients wonder why there must be any scar at all. My answer is that any time you cut through the skin, the skin will heal with a scar. My goal is to make the scar as invisible as possible. The best cosmetic result usually calls for a good surgeon, a good patient—and good luck.

Wounds heal rapidly, usually in a week or two. Depending on where the tumor is located, the stitches may remain in place for as little as 4 days (on the face) to as long as 2 weeks (if the cancer is located on the trunk). The patient is usually instructed to keep the wound dry during this time. The patient's activity is reduced for about 3 weeks, as it takes that long for a wound to reach 70% of its strength.

The specimen bottle is sent to the laboratory, where tissue is examined microscopically to see whether any of the edges of the skin are invaded by the skin cancer. If the specimens indicate that the tumor extends to its borders, then it is assumed that cancer still remains in the patient. Additional surgery is required. Usually, this is the point at which it is ideal for Mohs micrographic surgery to be used.

Advantages

Surgical excision has several advantages. Cure rate is high, and in some cases, the scar is hardly noticeable. Unlike some other forms of treatment, tissue is examined to see whether all the tumor has been removed—a good safety precaution. In addition, the entire procedure can be performed in one stage, while other types of treatment, such as chemotherapy and radiation, may require many sessions.

Disadvantages

One disadvantage of the technique is that a good deal of normal tissue is removed, leaving a wound larger than would otherwise be the case. A second disadvantage is that in certain areas, such as the scalp and forehead, the wound edges are difficult to pull back together. Finally, this technique requires considerable skill, surgical training, and experience.

Recommendations

Skin cancers best suited to this type of treatment are tumors located where there is abundant skin so that the opening can be easily sutured and closed.

In surgical excision of malignant melanoma, a much wider border of skin is usually taken around the tumor, and this often necessitates a skin graft rather than the simple wound closure described above.

RADIATION THERAPY

Two types of radiation are most often used to treat skin cancer: conventional x-rays and the electron beam.

Radiation therapy is usually reserved for elderly patients who are too ill to undergo surgery or who refuse to have it performed. It may also be used to treat very large cancers where reconstruction would be difficult. Short-term cosmetic results can be good, especially when the treated area is small. It should never be used on skin that has already suffered radiation damage and it is rarely used in younger patients.

Technique

The area to be irradiated is first outlined. Then a radiation beam is directed at the outlined area. The healthy tissue around it is usually protected with a lead shield. The treatment usually consists of several exposures, so the patient must return for at least three or four and possibly as many as 15 or more visits.

Advantages

Radiation is essentially painless and within the first 2 or 3 years cosmetic results are usually superior to those obtained by other techniques. The cure rate is high.

Disadvantages

There are several unique disadvantages. First, if radiation is used in a hairy area, it will produce permanent hair loss. Second, the radiation itself may cause skin cancers. Third, the patient must return for many visits. Fourth, the cosmetic results in the very long term are often inferior to those after treatment by other methods.

Recommendations

Radiation therapy should be used only when other methods are ruled out. Since undesirable long-term after-effects are common, only in very special cases should radiation therapy be used on patients under the age of 25.

CURETTAGE-ELECTRODESICCATION

Electrosurgery combined with curettage is a popular method of destroying skin carcinomas. Part of the process is electrodesiccation, in which high-frequency current is applied to the lesion, destroying tissue by "drying it out." Combining this process with curettage—scraping away the tissue with a curette—has proven highly effective in eradicating both precancerous and cancerous skin growths.

Electrosurgery with curettage is frequently used to treat smaller basal and squamous cell carcinomas, as well as certain keratoacanthomas and some cases of Bowen's disease. It is also used to treat other precancerous conditions such as leukoplakia and keratoses of all types. If leukoplakia is suspected, a biopsy should be done to confirm the diagnosis before treatment. The white patches may have developed into an invading squamous cell carinoma for which other forms of therapy are required.

Technique

A local anesthetic is injected under the skin. Once the area is numb, the surgeon uses a curette to scrape the soft, cancerous tissue off the remaining skin. Then an electric needle is used to burn a narrow border over the curetted site to ensure that it has been completely destroyed. By repeating the procedure two or three times, usually during one visit, the surgeon can, in many instances, destroy all of the diseased tissue.

There is little bleeding with this method. Usually the patient is advised to use a simple dressing for a few days, sometimes with an antibiotic ointment beneath the dressing. The wound requires more time to heal after electrosurgery than after excisional surgery, usually 2–4 weeks. Postoperative complications are relatively rare.

Advantages

This process is much simpler than excisional therapy and

can also be performed under local anesthesia in the physician's office. Suture removal is not necessary. In the hands of an experienced physician, the cure rate is 85%–95%.

Disadvantages

The main disadvantage of curettage-electrodesiccation is that the cosmetic results are not as good as those resulting from excisional surgery. Most doctors recommend that other techniques be used to remove growths on the face in the areas of the nose, mouth, and eyelids. Although in time the scars left by curettage-electrodesiccation become less conspicuous, they will always remain lighter in color than the surrounding skin.

Occasionally, enlarged scars (hypertrophic scars) or very rarely keloids will appear at the treated site. The thickened scars usually subside by themselves in time. Sometimes cortisone injections can hasten this shrinking process. Keloids are more difficult to eradicate. Some positive results have been reported by treating them with repeated injections of steroids, incisional or excisional surgery, radiation therapy, cryotherapy, or a combination of these methods.

Recommendations

This method is ideal for treating small lesions, or for many lesions on the body. It can usually be done in the physician's office in a very short period of time and has a cure rate of 85%–90% for primary lesions. Curettage-electrodesiccation is especially appropriate for removing growths on the scalp because the scar is usually invisible in the patient's hairline.

CRYOSURGERY

In cryosurgery, tissue is destroyed by freezing to -40°C or below. The cryogen (refrigerant) used today in cancer treatment is liquid nitrogen, the only cryogen effective in destroying malignant and premalignant skin tumors.

Technique

The tissue to be frozen usually consists of the entire growth and a margin of healthy tissue surrounding it. After the tumor is outlined, a spray gun is filled with liquid nitrogen and the nozzle held at a distance from the skin determined by the size of the area to be sprayed. The area is sprayed for about 30 seconds, then thawed for 2–5 minutes. This quick-freeze, slow-thaw cycle is repeated at least twice. The frozen area should not be covered by a dressing.

Results are not immediately apparent because it takes at least 24 hours for the tissue to die. At that time, the dead tissue looks very different from the living tissue. During the next few weeks the dead tissue sloughs off by itself, revealing a smooth pink surface that may remain swollen for several days.

There is no pain after the skin is completely frozen. However, there is sometimes intense pain during the procedure and afterwards, when the skin thaws. Local anesthetics may be needed before the operation and analgesics (painkillers) following it. This is essentially a bloodless procedure.

Advantages

The technique is quick and inexpensive. Cure rates are high. Best of all, the cosmetic results are good (although often not quite as good as with excisional surgery). Scarring is minimal.

Disadvantages

A disadvantage is the swelling and pain that exists during the first 24 hours after treatment. Furthermore, an open wound develops after treatment that often takes 4–6 weeks or more to heal.

Frequently there is a permanent loss of pigmentation, and when there is treatment over hair-bearing skin, hair will not regrow.

Recommendations

Primary basal cell carcinomas with well-defined borders respond well to this technique. The technique is also used in those patients who have many small skin cancers.

CHEMOTHERAPY

Chemotherapy for skin cancer includes the use of chemicals applied to the tumor itself (topical therapy) and the administration of chemicals in pills or by injection (systemic therapy).

Topical Therapy

The chemical 5-fluorouracil (5-FU) has been applied directly to the skin to treat small superficial basal cell carcinomas. However, this treatment has met with mixed success. To date the FDA has approved 5-FU only for treatment of solar keratoses, against which it has usually proven very effective. Other cancerous conditions, such as

Bowen's disease and superficial basal cell carcinoma located on the trunk, have been treated on a trial basis with 5-FU. The results have been variable. Some growths, particularly small ones, have been completely eliminated by treatment, while others seem barely affected.

Technique

A liquid or ointment form of the chemical is gently rubbed into the diseased tissue twice a day over a period ranging from 2 to 4 weeks for solar keratoses and 3 to 6 or even 12 weeks for superficial carcinomas. Pain, itching, and inflammation are quite variable from person to person. Some patients do not experience any discomfort, while others have such intense pain that they are unable to continue the treatment (this may be an allergic response).

5-Fluorouracil seems to have little or no effect on normal skin, attacking only the diseased tissues. Side effects are infrequent but, on the rare occasions when they do occur, can be severe. They include allergic dermatitis (an inflammation of the skin), soreness, swelling, scaling, and distended blood vessels.

Patients who have been treated with 5-FU are advised to stay out of the sun because ultraviolet light seems to encourage or enhance severe response.

Actually, the tendency of these growths to recur is greater after 5-FU treatment than after a more drastic approach. Yet the treatment is so simple and the cosmetic benefit so great (there is seldom any scarring) that in some cases both patient and doctor are willing to repeat the treatment periodically rather than resort to surgery, even if the cure by surgery is more likely to be complete.

Recommendations

Although topical chemotherapy cannot at this point be widely used for skin cancers, it is the best treatment for many precancerous conditions such as solar keratoses.

Systemic Therapy

In systemic chemotherapy, the prescribed chemical is either taken orally or injected into a vein or muscle rather than being applied to the skin. The method is called systemic because a large portion of the chemical circulates throughout the body. Generally, systemic chemotherapy is used only after other types of treatment have failed because many of the drugs can have harmful effects. Those drugs most frequently employed fall into the following basic groups: antimetabolites, alkylating agents, alkaloids, antibiotics, enzymes, biologic modifiers, and hormones. The cure rate is lower than with most other types of treatment.

Side effects are the rule rather than the exception and may include nausea, diarrhea, chills and fever, loss of hair, thickening and darkening of the skin, bone marrow depression (lowered capacity to produce blood cells), liver and kidney damage, and respiratory disorders, which may rarely be fatal.

Systemic chemotherapy is often used in the treatment of malignant melanoma and is discussed in detail in Chapter 21, Promising Research in Malignant Melanoma.

LASER THERAPY

Surgery by laser is a new technique that has shown some very promising results. A carbon dioxide (CO_2) laser is the one that is used mostly for cancer surgery. This apparatus permits the physician to work in one of two ways. The CO_2

laser can be used to evaporate tissue from the skin surface, or to excise tissue in its cutting mode, in which the beam will cut through tissue without bleeding. The laser can also can be used to cut bone without bleeding. Hence, it has advantages in patients who are taking blood thinners, by reducing the possibility of hemorrhaging.

Advantages and Disadvantages

The advantage of laser therapy is that it can be used on patients in very poor health. The disadvantages are that it is very time consuming, the equipment is extremely costly, and it is not readily available.

15

THE HEALING PROCESS: After Skin Cancer Treatment

*T*reatment does not end when your skin cancer has been removed. Your physician will consider both medical and cosmetic factors in choosing the best technique for closing and repairing wounds left after cancer treatment. The choice may be to let your wound heal naturally, to close it with stitches, or, if surgery has been extensive, to cover the area with a graft of skin from an adjacent or other part of your body. After that, your physician will want to see you for regular follow-up visits for several years to observe the site and be sure your cancer has not recurred.

The size of the growth is one factor determining healing. Even more important, though, is whether the growth was a first-time malignancy (primary lesion, no previous treatment) or one that recurred or persisted in the same location after initial cure (recurrent lesion). Recurrences coming from a previously treated site can be masked by a skin graft, skin flap, or even by closing of the wound with stitches, making them much harder to eradicate than a primary lesion. For this reason, before repairing the wound, the surgeon may wait a week or so for a report from a pathologist stating that no tumor cells remain.

Reconstructive surgery (surgery to correct large defects with skin grafts or skin flaps) may be delayed even longer. Because most recurrences occur in the first year after treatment, surgeons may wait as long as a year before reconstructing large defects to be sure that no persistent tumor remains. With extensive repairs, it is very difficult to detect residual cancer cells and determine whether they are growing inwardly. Frequently, prior to a repair additional biopsies are taken to ensure a field free of tumor cells.

PRIMARY CLOSURE: STITCHING THE WOUND

Primary closure means that the cut edges of an incision or wound are joined with stitches (sutures) or staples. It is the preferred method for small wounds in locations such as the cheek, the neck, and other areas where loose skin can be pulled together. Excellent cosmetic results are achieved; after a period of only 1–2 weeks, the stitches are removed. Within 4–5 weeks, usually only a linear scar is apparent. Scars over such areas of tension, such as shoulders and backs of legs, will stretch.

SPONTANEOUS HEALING

In many cases, the physician will decide to allow the wound to heal by itself after the cancer has been eradicated.

This method, which is not used often enough, has significant advantages. In spontaneous healing, the wound edges remain separate, the wound naturally fills with a substance called granulation tissue, and new skin grows over the area. Granulation tissue, or "proud flesh," is composed of blood vessels and fibrous tissue. Sometimes, it grows above the level of the surrounding surface skin, forming a scaffolding over which tissue from wound margins can grow. Depending on the wound size, this process can last 2 weeks to 6 months. The resulting scar is smooth and initially bright red. The color gradually fades to pink, then to near flesh tone. Although complete healing by this method may take as long as 1–2 months, the cosmetic results are often good.

Until recently, many physicians, including plastic surgeons, have had little or no experience with spontaneous healing (also called epithelialization). The surgical dictum that large wounds be immediately covered is too often followed. However, wounds often look better when allowed to heal naturally. In the concave areas around the nose and eyes, spontaneous epithelialization often provides the most acceptable cosmetic result.

Spontaneous healing has another great advantage: if the cancer recurs, it can be more readily identified and re-treated than if reconstructive surgery had been performed.

RECONSTRUCTIVE SURGERY

The need for reconstructive surgery depends on the size, nature, and site of the growth (the defect after the cancer is removed), as well as the number of previous attempts to remove the cancer and the types of treatment previously used. The physician who removes the growth may also perform the reconstructive surgery or may refer the patient to another surgeon specializing in the type of repair necessary.

In selected cases where there have been many recurrences,

it is not uncommon to delay reconstructive surgery for 12 months following treatment, a high-risk period when cancerous growths are most likely to recur. Exceptions are made in cases in which immediate reconstruction is needed to protect and shield vital organs, such as the eyelids to protect the cornea of the eye; or when the wound is in the area of the mouth, to permit the patient to eat and speak; and for professional reasons, when the patient cannot carry on work without cosmetic repair.

Today, the waiting period prior to reconstruction for such cases has been shortened for two reasons. First, the more difficult cases are being referred for treatment by Mohs surgery. This technique has a 93%–97% cure rate for recurrent lesions, making the risk of additional recurrence small. Second, the more difficult and complex cases are done in the operating room with surgical borders monitored through frozen sections examined by a pathologist at the time of surgery. Nonetheless, most surgeons will still elect to wait 6–12 months for reconstructive surgery in cases where the cancer has recurred repeatedly or where the chance of recurrence is high.

A waiting period is also advisable with the more difficult, large cases because there is usually only one good chance to reconstruct a defect. If a recurrence should develop after reconstructive surgery, the patient is probably denied the best result because any subsequent surgery will not be as cosmetically acceptable. This is particularly true in repairs of the nose.

Grafts

A good choice for repair of fairly large wounds (1–2 inches or more) is a graft, a layer of tissue taken from another part of the body to repair a surgical defect. Around the eye or mouth, where undue distortion may inevitably result from spontaneous healing or from primary closure, a surgeon may choose to cover the defect with tissue grafts.

Grafts are referred to by their thickness: a full-thickness skin graft uses the full thickness of skin; a split-thickness graft uses only the upper portion of the skin. The most common donor sites used for grafts are the back of the ear (postauricular area), the front of the ear (preauricular area), and the area above the collar bone. Sometimes excess tissue of the upper eyelid is used for grafts in the peri-orbital (eye) area. The skin of the preauricular area is the best color match for the nose, where one-third of skin cancer occurs; skin behind the ear is the next best match. Because these areas are limited in size, however, the collar bone area is used for large defects.

After the tissue is removed, the edges of the donor site are sutured together, and the skin-grafted tissue placed over the surgical defect and tacked down with a number of fine stitches. A small amount of pressure is used to immobilize the new skin. It usually takes about 1–2 weeks for a new blood supply to become established in the grafted tissue. Although not all grafts "take," the success rate is extremely high, and the cosmetic result is often good to excellent. It is important that the patient not consume alcohol, smoke, or take aspirin during the time the graft is taking hold.

Flaps

Frequently, flaps are used to repair a defect. A skin flap is an area of adjacent skin that is rotated or advanced to cover the defect. This method has a high success rate and usually "takes" completely because an all-natural blood supply is brought into the new area. The same precautions — eliminating smoking, alcohol, and aspirin — must be followed. A disadvantage to this technique is that where the tissue is rotated to fill the defect, the initial planes of the tumor are disturbed and it can become difficult to determine the exact location of the tumor should a recurrence appear.

RETREATMENT: MORE DIFFICULT, LESS SUCCESSFUL

Previously untreated basal cell carcinomas which are treated by conventional methods (surgical excision, electrosurgery, radiation, and cryosurgery) have cure rates approaching 85%–95%. When these same methods are used to treat locally recurrent disease, the cure rates drop to about 50%–60%. This holds true whether the same method is used for each treatment or if a combination of methods is used. (Mohs micrographic surgery is far more effective in treating recurrent basal and squamous cell carcinomas, with a cure rate of 93%–97%.)

Retreatment is always a much more difficult process than the original procedure. The tumor is embedded in scar tissue and can extend deep into the subcutaneous tissue, muscle, and bone. To ensure complete removal of the cancer cells, a large cut that is both deep and wide has to be made.

In retreatment it is also more difficult for the physician to estimate the extent of tumor growth. The scar tissue prevents the upward migration of the malignant cells, forcing them to travel horizontally before they surface, often far beyond the original site of the growth. Sometimes, what appears to be a new growth proves to be an extension of an old one, requiring more complicated surgery than had been thought necessary at the preliminary examination. This is even more true where tumors are growing over cartilage and bone.

Deciding which is the best method of wound closure is not always easy. Each case is an individual therapeutic problem. Therefore, the doctor will choose the method that he or she believes is best for the patient and the one that will achieve a successful result.

SCARS: THEY'LL LOOK BETTER IN TIME

All surgery, whether for removal of a growth or for reconstruction, leaves a scar. Whenever the skin is cut, even by the most skilled surgeons, a scar results. If skin cancer is detected and treated while the lesion is small, the scar that results should be quite acceptable. At first, scars are red or purple and can be unusually sensitive to temperature extremes because the granulation tissue contains abundant blood vessels. Some patients experience much discomfort unless they are careful to stay away from extreme heat and cold. Eventually, this hypersensitivity will disappear.

After the wound has healed, scar tissue will become white and contain fewer blood vessels than the skin surrounding it. There may also be a persistent itching for a while because the new skin contains fewer oil glands than normal. However, this too will eventually pass, and in the meantime, itching may be alleviated by applying petroleum jelly, creams, or ointments to the site.

Most scars look their worst between 2 and 6 months following treatment and look best $1\frac{1}{2}$ to 2 years later. Usually, patients who are unhappy with cosmetic results at 2–6 months are later well satisfied. It is my experience that scars improve with time, and I recommend doing the minimum amount of correction over the maximum period of time.

FOLLOW-UP CARE

Cancerous and precancerous conditions may recur even when they appear to have been adequately treated. No failsafe method of treatment yet exists. A patient should continue to see the physician for follow-up care to make sure that the growth has not recurred and also to check for new skin cancer at other locations. When compared with the general population, patients who have had one skin tumor have a 40% greater risk of developing new tumors in the next 5 years.

The program recommended for most patients is a visit to the doctor 1 month after the treatment has been completed, with follow-up visits at 3-month intervals for 1 year. After that, if all is well, the patient will be asked to visit the doctor on a semiannual and then annual basis. The minimum recommended follow-up period is 5 years. These visits to the physician's office are essential since recurrent or new growths are not always evident to the patient.

CHAPTER

16

MOHS
SURGERY

M

ohs micrographic surgery (or, more simply, Mohs surgery) has the highest cure rate for primary basal cell and squamous cell carcinomas and is the treatment of choice for locally recurrent skin cancers, offering an average cure rate of 95%. Use of any other method to treat local recurrences achieves a cure rate of only 50%–60%.

Mohs surgery is unique in its precision. Instead of removing the whole clinically visible tumor and a large area of normal-appearing skin around it, the Mohs surgeon removes the minimum amount of healthy tissue and totally removes the cancer. Thin layers of tissue are systematically excised and examined under a microscope for malignant cells. When all areas of tissue are tumor-free, surgery is complete.

The technique has several major advantages. It preserves more normal tissue than any other method while at the same time allowing the surgeon to trace and eradicate areas of tumor that are invisible to the naked eye. Physicians using other techniques to treat skin cancer must make an educated guess as to how far the skin cancer grows outwardly and downwardly. The Mohs surgeon, after examining the tissue under a microscope, knows exactly how far the tumor extends. Mohs surgery is thus particularly suitable for the area around the eyes, and the nose, ears, and mouth, where the preservation of normal tissue is essential.

The procedure does not require general anesthesia, which permits its use on many patients who are poor candidates for conventional surgery. Since the mortality rate is almost nil, elderly patients in poor health can be treated safely. Most patients do not have to be hospitalized and can be managed on an outpatient basis. The surgery can usually be completed in half a day or less.

Mohs surgeons have developed skills in surgery, pathology, and dermatology to enable them to perform this new, highly demanding technique. Unfortunately, because there are only about 200 trained Mohs surgeons in the United States, fewer than 20% of all skin cancers today are treated with the Mohs technique. As more physicians are trained, the technique should become more widely available.

History

The technique was developed about 40 years ago by Frederic E. Mohs, M.D., Professor of Surgery at the University of Wisconsin in Madison. Originally, Dr. Mohs called the procedure "chemosurgery" (it is still sometimes referred to by this term) because he applied a chemical to the cancerous lesion to "fix" the tissue before surgically removing it. Later, when the technique was improved and chemicals were no longer required, it was renamed Mohs surgery or, more formally, Mohs micrographic surgery. Twenty years ago, a society was formed, and stringent requirements for training in the procedure were established. Twenty leading medical centers now have 1–2-year training programs for physicians. Dermatologists, otolaryngologists (doctors who specialize in treating diseases of the head and neck), and plastic surgeons can acquire such training.

TECHNIQUE

The physician makes a reference map of the whole area to be excised. A local anesthetic is then injected. This is followed by the use of a curette (a ring-like instrument that removes the tumor located on the surface) (Figure 16.1). As each section of tissue around the cancerous site is surgically removed (Figure 16.2), it is identified on the map by its corresponding number. The edges of the specimen are dyed blue and red to indicate its specific direction and geographic relation to the other sections—superiorly, inferiorly, medially, and laterally (north, south, east, west).

Sections of tissue are removed in stages, and sent to an on-site laboratory for slide preparation and study. As each section is microscopically examined by the Mohs surgeon, the location of malignant cells is marked in color on the original map of numbered sections and oriented exactly by the red and blue coding (Figure 16.3). If a specific section that has been removed shows evidence of malignancy, another section will be removed in the area where tumor remains (Figure 16.4). The procedures of excision, mapping, and evaluation are repeated as often as necessary until the cancerous tissue is completely eradicated. As few as one or two sections, or as many as a dozen or more, may be removed.

Most Mohs surgery cases are completed in only two or three stages, so the entire procedure is often finished in less than 2 hours (Figure 16.5).

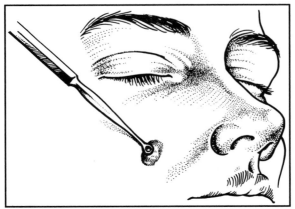

(Figure 16.1)
A curette is used to remove the tumor.

(Figure 16.2)
The tissue is surgically excised in thin layers and a map is prepared to show the location of the sections.

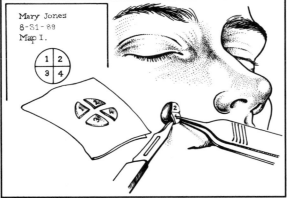

(Figure 16.3)
Microscopic slides are prepared and examined. Positive areas showing tumor are colored in the map.

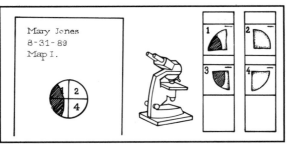

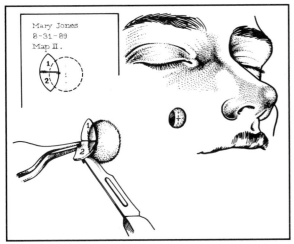

(Figure 16.4)
Additional tissue is surgically removed from the area showing tumor involvement.

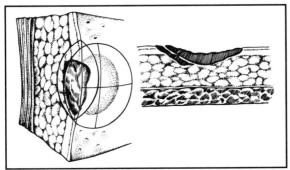

(Figure 16.5)
A cross-section of skin showing extension of tumor.

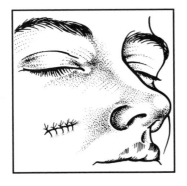

(Figure 16.6)
The wound is closed primarily.

If possible, the wound will be closed primarily (Figure 16.6). It also may be left to heal by itself, a process that normally takes an average of 4–8 weeks. Or it may be repaired with a skin flap or skin graft. Usually the repair will be discussed with the patient, who will be asked to restrict physical activity for a day or so and will be taught how to change the dressing on the wound.

The scar that is left after healing, as discussed earlier, can be corrected at a later date, if necessary. The body does a wonderful job of improving scars with time. Therefore, I repeat, it is often recommended to do the minimum correction over the maximum period of time.

ADVANTAGES

The advantages of microscopically controlled surgery are unprecedented reliability, conservatism, low operative mortality, good healing without adverse side effects, and feasibility of the operation to many patients in poor health. Lastly, where other standard modalities have been unsuccessful, Mohs surgery offers a chance for cure.

DISADVANTAGES

Mohs surgery is not yet widely available. The American College of Mohs Micrographic Surgery, located in Evanston, Illinois, can provide a listing of Mohs surgeons who have met the requirements of specialized training before becoming eligible for membership in the Society. The Society has a toll-free number (1-800-441-2737) that is in effect between 9:00 am and 5:00 pm Central Time. During the past 24 years, I have personally trained 23 physicians who are now performing the technique in the United States and abroad.

C H A P T E R
17

CASE HISTORIES
CASE HISTORIES
CASE HISTORIES
MOHS
CASE HISTORIES
CASE HISTORIES
CASE HISTORIES
CASE HISTORIES
CASE HISTORIES

MOHS CASE
HISTORIES

*T*he following case histories are examples of extensive skin cancers in which Mohs surgery has been of great benefit. In most patients, skin cancer does not reach such extreme stages before being detected and does not involve extensive loss of tissue or of eye, ear, or nose. For skin cancers detected and treated promptly, treatment is simple and the resultant scar is minimal.

CASE 1

Within a 10-year period, a 50-year-old man had had 14 operations and skin grafts as well as x-ray and radium treatments for a basal cell carcinoma of the face. He had been hospitalized once or twice a year for treatment of his skin cancer.

He was referred for Mohs surgery. Very little tumor growth was apparent on the surface of the skin; however, as microscopically controlled surgery proceeded, tumor cells were evident everywhere in the specimen tissue. The patient was hospitalized for continued treatment, and a substantial amount of tissue on the left side of his face as well as his entire nose had to be removed. Reconstructive surgery was then done. The patient is now 61 and as of this date has not had a recurrence of skin cancer.

CASE 2

When a 21-year-old student first noticed an elevated red spot on her nose and visited a dermatologist, the spots were believed to be sebaceous cysts, benign cysts that arise from sweat glands. The lesions did not respond to injections but continued to grow. The dermatologist then referred her to a surgeon, who excised the growth. The pathology report showed it to be a basal cell carcinoma. She returned to school abroad, but after 1 month, another growth over the same spot appeared. On examination, it appeared small, but Mohs surgery showed it to be so extensive that it was necessary to remove most of her nose.

Because of the extent of the defect, the patient was at first severely depressed. However, with psychological help and skillful reconstructive surgery, she improved dramatically and has lived a happy, healthy life for the past 14 years. If this patient had been treated by standard surgical procedures, some of the cancer probably would have been missed, which could have threatened her life or caused great disfigurement.

CASE 3

For years, dentists have held a small film plate in their patients' mouths while they took x-ray films of the teeth.

This occupational exposure to radiation often resulted in cancer of the thumb or fingers. Injury to the thumb was more serious than that to the fingers because of the thumb's greater importance to dexterity and function of the hand.

A 67-year-old dentist had been treated for many years by a dermatologist in an effort to cure a radiation injury of his thumb. Eventually, the condition deteriorated, and a biopsy showed skin cancer. The dentist was then told by a hand surgeon that amputation would be necessary, but another physician suggested that he consult a Mohs surgeon. With Mohs surgery, the dentist's thumb was saved, and he did not lose a day's work.

Case 4

Skin cancers sometimes occur at the site of an injury. A 34-year-old man was found to have a basal cell carcinoma on an area near the eye that had been injured by a firecracker when he was a child. Initially, the malignancy was treated with x-ray therapy. Two years later, the cancer recurred and was treated with excision and grafting. A further recurrence in 1969, when the patient was 42 years old, was then treated by Mohs surgery. Microscopic examination at that time showed that the tumor had extended so far that the eye had to be removed. The cancer has not recurred in the 14 years since completion of Mohs surgery.

Case 5

Skin cancer can be hard to diagnose, especially when it has an atypical appearance. Physicians had told one patient that her red nose was probably caused by dilated veins.

Unconcerned, despite a family history of skin cancer and excessive sun exposure, she did not see a physician again until 2 years later, when the skin at the end of her nose began to bleed. Mohs surgery performed on this patient revealed basal cell carcinoma and resulted in removal of most of her nose. However, with reconstruction her appearance is now quite acceptable, and she has had no recurrence of the skin cancer.

SKIN CANCER PATIENTS TELL THEIR OWN STORIES

*O*f necessity, my primary focus as a physician is the clinical side of skin cancer: using the most sophisticated methods of dealing with each individual case in order to eliminate the disease with as little trauma as possible — and, in some cases, save the patient's life.

But I'm acutely aware of the vital human side of the story as well. Despite much progress in diagnosis and treatment, the emotional impact of skin cancer is still considerable. Here, five patients, three of them mine, share their various experiences fighting skin cancer. As each reveals, in his or her own words, the importance of sun protection and early detection had to be learned the hard way.

As Peter Ward discovered, no medical checkup is complete without a skin survey from head to toe.

In 1978, while I was living in Los Angeles, a friend of mine had a very serious malignant melanoma that required extensive surgery in his lower abdomen. He later stressed to me that I should have a skin examination as soon as possible, as the incidence of skin cancer was far greater than the public was aware of. In 1981, I had a complete annual physical exam at a well-known institution in New York that specializes in such checkups, and was disappointed to find there was no examination of my skin. When I mentioned this in my office, one of my partners suggested I could very easily have a complete skin cancer checkup done.

I proceeded to make an appointment with Dr. Perry Robins at New York University Medical Center. Dr. Robins examined my entire body and noticed a slight lesion on my lower leg that concerned him enough to do a biopsy. I had never noticed this lesion or had any irritation from it. In a matter of days, Dr. Robins called me and said I must come in immediately for surgery, as the laboratory had diagnosed malignant melanoma.

I had the surgery the following morning. In those few hours, I was shocked into the terrifying seriousness, the life and death implications, of what my friend had told me in California. I thank God and the alertness of my doctor for saving my life. As he and two other physicians made clear, it would have been only a matter of months before the melanoma would have spread out of control and possibly been terminal. And I had not even noticed the lesion.

At a fit 33, just promoted exec Barbara Boulware was feeling fine — until a mole went out of control.

On Easter Sunday, while basking in the spring sunshine, I confided to a friend that I wasn't looking forward to having the large mole on my back removed. After all, I'd had it all my life. But it had bled recently when I toweled off, so maybe it was a little irritated.

Little did I know that the next day the dermatologist would take one look at my back and call a surgeon; the surgeon would in turn declare, "I'm ninety-nine percent sure you have a malignant melanoma." He would place two hands on my back and say, "I'll have to take this much of your back in surgery. We'll operate Thursday." "Will I be okay after that?" I would ask incredulously. "We certainly hope so," would be his honest reply.

Still stunned, I entered the hospital to undergo the surgery necessary to save my life. My condition was confirmed as malignant melanoma — Clark level 3. The good news was that the cancer hadn't spread: my doctor was confident all of the cancer had been removed during surgery.

That Friday, the long process of healing — physically and mentally — began. For the next $2\frac{1}{2}$ weeks, I would call the hospital home. As with many advanced melanoma patients, a large skin graft was needed to heal the large wound on my back. The donor site on my derriere was very tender. Gradually, though, I began feeling better. Checking out of the hospital, I was ecstatic at the prospect of going home.

But my first visit back to the doctor was another shocker. My skin graft was not taking, and a second surgery was necessary. The tears I had so far refused to shed fell freely and effusively.

When my doctor at last announced on a Friday, "You can begin half days at work on Monday," I was terrified. How would people react to me? I walked into the office that Monday morning with a knot in my stomach tied with anxiety. However, after I had made those first few scary steps, I knew the final stages of healing had begun.

Sixteen-year-old Sandy Conlin is living proof that kids can get skin cancer, too.

It was just after I was back in school after a really fun summer at Cape Cod with my family that I noticed a sore that was beginning on the side of my nose where I had been sunburned and was peeling. At first I kind of ignored it, until it became bigger and wouldn't go away. It was crusty and oozing and really ugly. My mom thought it was that way because I was picking at it, even though I kept telling her that I wasn't. It just got worse, and finally she said I would have to go to the doctor right away to have it checked out.

She took me to a dermatologist, and he removed some of my tissue with a long needle to send to the lab for analysis. A few days later we found out I had something called basal cell carcinoma. Mom and Dad were shocked and really upset because they thought I was much too young to have skin cancer.

My mom took me to New York to Dr. Robins, and he told her that what appears to be on the surface of the skin does not tell you what is going on underneath. He did not want to alarm her, but he did tell her that he might have to go quite deep and wide to get all the cancer cells. You have to get all the cancer cells to make sure the cancer will not grow back. Then the body can repair itself with good healthy cells.

I had to go into surgery four times because the cancer cells just kept coming. Each time Dr. Robins removed a layer and the lab technician prepared it for the microscope. My mom and I looked at the slide under a special microscope so that we could see the healthy cells, which appeared a pinkish purple, and the cancer cells, which appeared black, irregular and rather grotesque.

I was left with a big hole in my nose. My parents decided

to let it heal as best it could and then consider plastic surgery if I needed it at a later time.

Dr. Robins gave me a little clear plastic case like a box in which there were little drawers, one each for the four slides. I brought them to school for my biology class to see. None of the kids had ever seen a cancer cell. One weekend, I went to a party, and everybody asked me a lot of questions. I really didn't want to talk about it, but I was glad I could make my friends aware that it could happen to them, too.

Inspired by fellow fighters, skin cancer patient Sharon Pratt came out on top and now gives others a helping hand.

I am a survivor of malignant melanoma. My cancer began in a mole on my back. Six months after it was removed, it spread to my lymph nodes; I was three months pregnant with my second child at the time. After my daughter was born, a tumor in my lung was diagnosed and removed. Since that time I have been a part of an experimental protocol aimed at preventing recurrence. So far, the treatment has been successful for me.

There are many things that have contributed to my recovery, but one in particular stands out: the love and support of other patients and survivors.

Hearing I had cancer changed every part of my life. It was a terrifying and isolating experience. Nobody knew how to help me. I remember Doris — she was the first survivor who reached out to me. She helped me in practical and spiritual ways that no one else could. This first experience of networking allowed me to see how important it is to connect with other people who share my hopes and fears.

After meeting other patients and their families while in

New York for treatment, I realized that we would all benefit from having a way to share information and support. What resulted is a newsletter called The Helping Hand and a network of close to 100 patients and survivors. The newsletter is a collection of articles and information about melanoma collected by the people in the network. It is a very "grassroots" operation — I cut and paste it in my kitchen. Despite its homespun qualities, it brings hope and inspiration to those who receive it. Through these connections we have been able to break down the walls of silence and isolation. We have all been able to find a strength inside ourselves that has helped us with our battles.

For former sun worshipper Jennie Caprio, the quest for the perfect tan meant devastating disfigurement.

My skin cancer first appeared in 1973 at the end of the summer. I noticed a tiny freckle on the left side of my nose that hadn't been there before. It was completely flat, and after a while it turned from light brown to black. I went to a doctor who looked at the spot and said, "I think it's skin cancer. You should have it removed."

Before I could get to a surgeon, the spot began to bleed. I was terrified, but the surgeon didn't explain anything to me. He strapped me onto a table, gave me shots in my nose of a local anesthetic, and started cutting out the spot. I went back a week later to have the bandage removed, and for the first time I saw I had a pea-sized indentation. The doctor told me he thought he had removed all the cancer. When I asked him about going in the sun, he said, "Don't get paranoid — just put some lotion on."

Since no one had said the sun was responsible for my cancer, I continued sunning myself. The cancer recurred in

1978. I went to a specialist who said he could get rid of the cancer through radiation. It was like getting an x-ray, but my nose began to look like it had a burn on it. It blistered and oozed. Finally, a scab formed and when that fell off, a white scar remained. The doctor told me to cover up in the sun, which I did.

On vacation in Arizona, I would sit under an umbrella with my hat on and zinc oxide all over me. One day I looked in the mirror and saw that the tip of my nose was livid. As distressed as I was, I didn't see a doctor right away. I guess I didn't want to know the truth.

When I got home 2 months later, I went to Dr. Robins, who explained that I had basal cell carcinoma, caused by years of exposure to the sun. He said he would remove the cancer using the Mohs technique.

He gave me a shot in my nose to deaden the pain and then took the first slice from the tip. That happened three more times. I didn't look at myself, but under the bandage I could feel that my nose was getting flatter. But it wasn't until 2 months after surgery that I looked at my nose for the first time. My first reaction was, "Oh, my God!" Then I decided not to let it get me down. By that time, I was using skin-toned bandages, and I always made sure the rest of me looked perfect.

I had always planned to have reconstructive surgery, and 10 months later Dr. Robins said I was ready. I went to Dr. Daniel Baker, a Manhattan plastic surgeon, who at first was reluctant to do it. He explained that they usually take skin from the forehead to graft onto the nose, but that because my forehead was small, it presented a problem. I explained to him that I didn't expect miracles. Despite the problems my case presented, he agreed to do the surgery.

The reconstruction was done in two steps. The first involved bringing the front of my scalp forward and attaching a patch of skin from the side of my forehead to my nose. It had to stay like that for about two weeks, in order to allow the blood vessels to begin regenerating. Then they replaced the skin that had been taken from my forehead with a skin graft from behind my ear. Despite the pain, I recovered quickly and 10 days later went home from the hospital. My nose was swollen, but it was okay. It was a nose.

In the past few years, I've had several more operations, mostly to reduce the visible scars. I never sit in the sun anymore. If I go out, I always wear sunblock, a hat, and long sleeves. I lecture everyone about the sun's dangers, but it's hard to get the message across. They often say what I said when I first learned I had it: "Skin cancer? What's that?"

CHAPTER
19

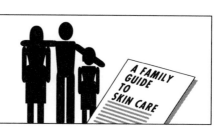

FAMILY SKIN CARE: A Guide Through the Years

I f you've absorbed the message of this book, you know by now that skin protection is crucial for every member of your family. In the youngest, you'll want to establish good habits and, as a parent, set the best possible example. For teens, who may be more concerned with their friends than with possible skin cancer decades later, you'll need to use patience and ingenuity. As an adult moving toward the danger years when cumulative skin damage results in skin cancer, you'll want to continue good sun protection practices—or develop new ones—and be vigilant for suspicious lesions. You also may want a little advice about keeping your skin looking as young as possible.

This chapter contains sun protection guidance for different age groups as well as help for some common skin problems.

GUIDELINES FOR THE WHOLE FAMILY
Studies show that habitual use of a sunscreen with a sun

protection factor of 15 during the first 18 years of life can reduce the lifetime incidence of non-melanoma skin cancer by 78%. For the average child who has skin that tans fairly easily, who lives in an average northern summer climate, and who has average sun-seeking behavior, the cost of a sunscreen from birth to age 18 is approximately $310—about $17 yearly or only 5 cents per day!

Your whole family should follow these simple guidelines to protect themselves from the sun's damaging rays:

1. Avoid peak hours of sunlight (10:00 am to 3:00 pm).
2. Wear protective clothing.
3. Use a sunscreen of SPF #15 or higher.
4. Teach children sun protection early in life.
5. Do not work on a tan.
6. Do not patronize tanning salons.
7. Examine your skin regularly.
8. If you notice any changes, see your physician promptly.

SKIN CARE: INFANCY TO ADOLESCENCE

Newborn skin is healthy skin. Children's skin is usually just about as healthy as it looks—smooth, glowing, and resilient. Your job as a parent is to keep it that way. From infancy through the childhood years, it is the parents' responsibility to protect young skin, to establish good skin care habits, and, in older children, to supervise.

Sensitive Skin

A child's skin, particularly type I or II, is far more sensitive than adult skin because the stratum corneum, or outermost horny layer of skin, is thinner. Moreover, as children we spend triple the amount of time in the sun that we do as adults. Most sun damage occurs between the ages of 5 and 15 and can have a major influence on the development of skin cancer later in life. Therefore, protection of children's skin is crucial.

A common misconception is that young skin, which regenerates faster than adult skin, can take sun insult and heal itself. Although it is true that sunburns usually heal with minimal or no scarring, latent damage remains.

Caring for Younger Skin

Generally, follow the family guidelines outlined above. You can usually start using a sunscreen when your infant is about 6 months old. Before that time, the baby should not be exposed to the sun.

Cover as much as possible of your infant's or toddler's skin with protective clothing. Use wide-brimmed hats and strollers and carriages that have protective canopies and hoods. (Remember that these do not provide complete protection from ultraviolet rays.)

When you begin to use sunscreen on your child, choose a non-alcohol-based product, and even then, try to take your child outdoors only before 10 am or after 3 pm. Take extra care if there is a family history of skin cancer and/or your child's skin is very fair. Make application of sunscreen a daily routine, especially in the summer. Apply it when changing diapers, for example, or just before snack time. Be sure to choose a water-resistant variety when your toddler is paddling in the water.

If your child attends a day care center, nursery school, or kindergarten, let the school personnel know when a sunscreen should be used; be sure to pack it in the school bag, and let the staff know where it is.

Finally, when you bathe and care for your child, become aware of the normal appearance of the child's skin. If any new growth appears or change occurs, consult your pediatrician or dermatologist.

The School-Age Child

In the school-age child, see to it that sun protection becomes a habit—like toothbrushing or hair combing. Your child is more independent now but needs your help and reminders about sun protection just the same. Be sure the sunscreen used is SPF 15 or higher. Pack a tube in his or her overnight bag when visiting friends.

Your school-age child will spend many hours outside your direct supervision. Be sure teachers, gym instructors, and camp counsellors know your child should be using a sunscreen, why, and how to apply it. Do not use tanning lotions and baby oil; these will only make your child burn more easily.

If your child does become sunburned, treat the condition immediately. Here are some things you can do to ease the associated pain and discomfort:

1. Soothe sunburned skin with wet compresses of cool tap water or 1:40 Burow's solution for 20 minutes, 3–4 times a day. Wet compresses help dull the pain and reduce redness and swelling.

2. Coat the sunburned area with a lubricating lotion (such as baby lotion) or cream to relieve some of the dryness and help promote healing. Avoid heavy, greasy emollients.

3. Use pain relievers, such as acetaminophen, as needed.

4. Have your child drink plenty of water to replace lost fluids.

5. Do not allow your child any more sun exposure until the skin has healed completely. Sunburned skin can take up to several days to repair, and skin that is already burned is more susceptible to a second burn.

If blistering or oozing develops, consult your pediatrician or dermatologist promptly.

Adolescence

It is hard if not impossible to persuade a reluctant teenager to apply sunscreen regularly. My two teenagers, with a father who is a specialist in skin cancer, have made minimal concessions to using sunscreens because they were usually actively pursuing a tan. However, in the last year or two, their friends have been using a sunscreen with an SPF of 15, and they are now experimenting with sunscreens with a higher SPF.

Your teen should be following the same guidelines as the rest of the family. But don't let sun protection become a battleground. If good habits have been established, your child has already enjoyed years of protection and will probably return to good habits when the rebellious adolescent years have passed.

If sun protection is new to your teen, be sure he or she understands why you think sun protection is important. Remind your teenager that more sun time may be accumulated than realized, in washing a car, doing lawn chores, and participating in school outdoor activities.

Always be prepared to compromise. If your adolescent won't wear an SPF of 15, settle for slightly less protection; if a hat is not in style, buy that funky visor everyone else is wearing that year.

ACNE: ROLE OF SUNLIGHT

Whether sunlight benefits or threatens acne patients is not clear. For years, physicians and patients have noticed that acne improved during the summer months, when exposed to more sunlight. Ultraviolet rays are used by some doctors to treat acne. Others contend that the summer improvement in acne is only cosmetic—blemishes are less apparent against a tanned skin.

Some dermatologists believe that sunlight offers more than cosmetic benefit, somehow modulating inflammation. Others believe that the lessened stress that coincides with summer vacation is the true, if temporary, skin healer. Still others strongly believe that the sun will worsen acne.

Acne patients need not resign themselves to a sunless life until the causes of acne are understood and adequate treatment is available.

Here are some guidelines to follow if you have acne:

1. Use a water-resistant, noncomedogenic (non-pore-blocking) sunscreen that is not oily, such as an alcohol-based sunscreen that has a sun protection factor of 15 or more.

2. Apply acne medication before applying sunscreen, either in the evening or early morning before sun exposure, being sure to reapply sunscreen after swimming or perspiring heavily or in humid weather.

3. Consult with your physician about possible interactions between acne medications (especially antibiotics), astringents, deodorant or antiseptic soaps and lotions, and sunscreens and sunlight.

ADULT SKIN: THE AGING PROCESS

Skin does not suddenly begin to age as we reach midlife.

Aging is ongoing—and there are actually two processes: photoaging, which begins at birth, is primarily due to sun exposure, and is cumulative; and biological aging, which is a naturally occurring inherent process that may become evident as early as age 30 in some individuals. The skin of the more exposed areas of the body, the face and backs of the hands, photoages earliest. The eyelids, where the skin is only one millimeter thick, especially show the effect of aging more rapidly. The effects of habitual expressions, the register of our emotions by the many facial muscles, begin to show lines, grooves, puckers, and creases—the permanent result of smiles, frowns, tension, and stress.

The epidermis dries as the function of the sweat glands decreases, and cell regeneration and replacement slows. Sun exposure damages the melanin-producing cells, causing blotches, commonly called "age" or "liver" spots. Lack of moisture and oil causes dryness and wrinkles. Cell build-up occurs at the surface, resulting in uneven pigmentation.

In the dermis, collagen begins to decrease and tangle, a condition called solar elastosis. There is a concomitant loss of fat cells. Owing to all these factors, the skin is more fragile, susceptible to damage and easy bruising, and slower to heal. These changes in texture, color, and contour, at first almost imperceptible, are usually readily apparent as early as age 25 in those exposed to solar radiation. Although it is a biological inevitability that we will age, wrinkle, and sag somewhat with the years, and although the amount we experience is influenced by genes and the geographical area we inhabit, we can control to a degree the amount of wrinkling the skin undergoes by practicing sun avoidance.

How much of these combined effects are caused by the sun and how much by age itself? Sun effects can be seen by comparing the skin on the face and backs of the hands with the skin on a part of the body that is seldom exposed, such as the buttocks. These effects are also apparent in the leathery skin of outdoor workers, in contrast to the smooth unlined skin of people in cultures and societies that practice sun avoidance.

As an adult, continue good sun-protection practices. At this time of life, you'll want to be especially alert for early signs of skin cancer. For this reason, a total body skin examination should be performed at least every 6 months. If you are in a high-risk group, the exam should be done every month or as often as your physician dictates.

LOOKING GOOD: HELP FOR THE AGING SKIN

A number of methods are available to help erase the damaging effects of aging.

Chemical Peel

Chemical peel, in which a caustic agent is applied to a small area, or more commonly, to the entire face and neck, is one method used for removal of scarring caused by acne, fine lines, and cross-hatching. Severe inflammation results, and for several weeks the region crusts and oozes, then the old skin sloughs off. The new skin is smooth and fine-pored—very cosmetically acceptable. However, side effects can occur, depending on the type of peel performed, skin coloring, and the previous condition of the skin. The results of a chemical peel are most noticeable where there has been extensive skin damage with many wrinkles or a leathery texture. The lasting benefit depends on the quality of the skin, the person's age, and general health. Local anesthesia is used. The amount of pain experienced varies.

Dermabrasion

Dermabrasion, a gentler process, is accomplished by a high-speed rotary wheel or disc of sandpaper, or a wire brush that planes either small or large areas of skin to a smooth surface. It is a method frequently used for removing fine lines around the mouth or eyes and for pitting or minor scarring, stimulating skin cells to regenerate. As with chemical peel, a crust forms and sloughs off within weeks to reveal the new, close-textured skin.

Facelifts and Other Surgical Procedures

In a total facelift, the entire skin is separated from the underlying tissue. Excess skin is cut away, and the remainder is repositioned and recontoured. Usually the neck area is included. This surgery often requires general anesthesia and involves the potential of nerve damage. Deep folds and wrinkles cannot be eliminated entirely, but the cosmetic appearance is usually dramatically improved.

Chinlifts, ear tucks, fat reductions, and lifts in almost all body areas can be readily accomplished today. Often these procedures alleviate physical and psychological distress and are eminently beneficial. Nonetheless, any surgery carries risks and potential for serious damage to nerves and internal organs. The surgical process is costly and temporary, with effects lasting from 6 to 10 years. Repeated surgery may result in a masklike appearance, and no surgery will correct underlying associated emotional problems or restore lost youth. Finally, and most important, any surgical process requires the skilled hands and knowledge of a qualified surgeon.

Retin-A

Retin-A creams are being used and studied widely as a treatment for sun-damaged skin, particularly the fine wrinkling caused by sun exposure over many years. As of now, the drug is only approved by the FDA for use in the treatment of a skin condition called acne vulgaris; it has not been approved for the general public for treating sun-damaged skin. The results of studies performed at different research centers on the effects of Retin-A on sun-damaged skin will be presented to the FDA. Whether the drug will be approved for this purpose is not yet known.

When used over a period of 4 to 22 months, Retin-A seems to significantly improve the fine wrinkles on sun-damaged skin. This effect seems to become stronger the longer the creams are used. Also, rough skin, sagging skin around the eyes, and liver spots can often be improved.

There are some drawbacks. Retin-A creams are very irritating, especially around the eyes and mouth, where their cosmetic effect is most wanted. As a result, Retin-A is usually first used in a low dosage form; it is gradually applied more often and at higher concentrations until the patient can no longer tolerate its irritating effects. People with very severe, sensitive, or painful irritations are sometimes advised to use the cream less often. Old or sun-damaged skin may be less sensitive to these irritations. However, the skin becomes accustomed to the drug over a period of weeks or months. If use of the cream is discontinued, part of the cosmetic effect is lost.

Retin-A creams can cause reddening and scaling of solar keratoses, the dry, scaly lesions that sometimes develop into squamous cell carcinoma. However, its effectiveness in treating these precancerous growths has yet to be proven. As with all medications, it is essential that Retin-A be used only under physician supervision.

It is important to note that the cosmetic effect of Retin-A —reduced wrinkles and lines—varies widely among people and does not occur rapidly. Treatment must be maintained over a period of months before any significant changes are observed. The effect of the creams on wrinkles caused by sun exposure and those due to natural aging are very different. At this point, sun-damaged skin seems to respond better to treatment.

While Retin-A creams can improve lines and wrinkles, they also make skin even more sensitive to the effects of the sun. People who use these creams must apply a sunscreen with a protection factor of at least 15 if they are going to spend time outdoors, and they should avoid any direct exposure to ultraviolet radiation. If sunbathing is an important part of your life, you probably should not use Retin-A.

C H A P T E R

20

TOTAL
BODY
SKIN
EXAMINATION

Because early detection and diagnosis of skin cancer is critical to its cure, I advocate a regular total body skin exam. Knowledge of your own skin—its normal pigmentation, imperfections, growths, and moles—permits you to quickly spot any change (see chart). A physician is the best person to determine whether that change warrants biopsy or treatment.

A total body skin examination should cover all areas of the skin from head to foot. It requires a few simple household tools and objects (as shown in Figures 20.1 to 20.3), a well-lit room, and careful scrutiny. It is briefly and easily accomplished.

I recommend that everyone, including children over 4, perform such an examination at least once every 6 months. A professional exam should be done yearly, as part of your annual medical checkup. Persons at high risk for skin cancer should examine themselves at least once a month and have themselves checked professionally every 6 months, or as often as the physician recommends.

SELF-CHECK CHART: MOLES

Moles larger than three millimeters in diameter are the most likely to cause trouble. A yearly check recorded on this chart can spot changes early.

MEASUREMENT GUIDE

3mm	5mm	7mm	9mm	11mm	13mm	15mm

GETTING TO KNOW YOUR SKIN: WHAT'S NORMAL

Most of us have a number of moles and blemishes on our skin; some have hundreds of hypo- or hyperpigmented areas, warts, skin tags, or other small skin imperfections. For the most part, they are insignificant, neither alarming nor threatening, and of cosmetic consideration only. Descriptions of some frequently found blemishes are given below.

Cherry Hemangiomas

Small bright red pimples, bumps, or purplish blotches, called cherry hemangiomas, may be almost invisible or as large as an eighth of an inch. They occur most commonly on the trunk and may appear in large numbers in early adulthood.

Lentigines

Lentigines, often called "age" spots or "liver" spots (because of their brown color), are commonly seen on the sun-exposed skin of 85% of elderly persons. The spots are the result of excess sun damage, however, and not of age. They result from uneven clustering of melanocytes in response to sunlight. Lentigines are light or dark brown flat areas. Although unattractive, they are harmless.

Spider Hemangiomas

Spider hemagiomas are the bright red tracery of blood capillaries often evident on the legs and thighs and on the noses of heavy drinkers. These red vessels also appear on the skin of the elderly.

WHAT TO WATCH FOR

Watch for any of these signs of skin cancer:

• A skin growth that increases in size and appears pearly, translucent, tan, brown, black, or multicolored.

• A mole, birthmark, or beauty mark that: changes color, increases in size or thickness, changes in texture, is irregular in outline.

• A spot or growth that continues to itch, hurt, crust, scab, erode, or bleed.

• An open sore or wound on the skin that does not heal or persists for more than 4 weeks, or heals and then reopens.

If you note any of skin cancer's warning signs, remember the following:

DON'T overlook it.

DON'T irritate it with tight clothing, straps, belt, shoe, etc.

DON'T aggravate it by picking, scratching, soaking, or applying a topical medication.

DON'T delay—consult your physician.

TOTAL BODY SKIN EXAMINATION: HOW IT'S DONE

The skin examination is best performed immediately after you have bathed or showered. You will need a good light, two chairs or stools, two mirrors, one full-length and one hand-held mirror, and a blow-dryer (Figures 20.1 through 20.3). For skin areas that are difficult for you to see yourself, you may need the assistance of a family member or friend.

The entire procedure will require about 10 minutes. Begin by examining your hands thoroughly: palms, backs, the fingernails, and between the fingers. Examine your wrists and forearms, front and back. Standing in front of the full-length mirror, hold your arms up and examine inner arms and armpits. Remember, you are learning the normal condition of your skin so that you will be aware of future change. Therefore, be aware of the skin tone and general pigmentation as well as freckles, beauty marks, moles, and skin tags.

Next, with your back to the full-length mirror, use the hand mirror to examine your upper back and the backs of your upper arms. Next examine your neck and chest area. If you are a woman, examine your breasts carefully, including areas that may be subjected to pressure from straps or elastic bands.

Examine your face, particularly the rims and lobes of your ears, and your nose, lips, and mouth. Remember, 80% of skin cancers appear on the head and neck. Use the blow-dryer (cool setting) to part your hair section by section, examining your entire scalp. You may need assistance in this.

Examine your lower back, buttocks, and genital areas with the aid of both mirrors. While seated, prop up one leg at a time on the opposite chair or stool. Check the soles, toenails, between the toes, heels, ankles, shins, calves, and thighs.

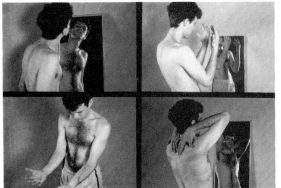

(Figure 20.1)
Examine your skin regularly. Inspect all areas of your body, including your head, neck, and arms.

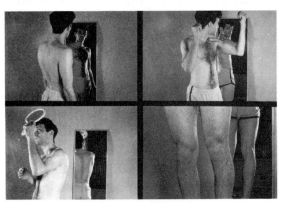

(Figure 20.2)
Also, don't forget to examine your front, sides, upper back, and lower body.

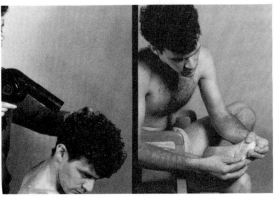

(Figure 20.3)
Use the blow-dryer to part your hair, section by section. Also, check your feet carefully.

Don't neglect any area. A total body skin examination performed regularly in this fashion will allow immediate detection of the slightest change in skin condition. If any change occurs, see a physician promptly.

PROFESSIONAL EXAMINATION

Ask your physician to perform a complete skin examination during your annual checkup. Little additional time will be required. Your physician is also trained to decide whether a lesion is suspicious, can advise you of the best treatments, and make referrals if needed.

COMMUNITY AND WORKPLACE EXAMINATIONS

Growing awareness of the need for and benefits of the total body skin examination has prompted The Skin Cancer Foundation, the American Academy of Dermatology, hospitals, health agencies, and individual employers to establish skin cancer detection and screening clinics. These provide much-needed information, examination, advice, and referrals. Such programs have revealed alarming numbers of previously undetected skin cancers, even in areas of high socioeconomic standards and easy access to medical care.

In a recent New York metropolitan area study, for example, 290 cases of early skin cancer, including 14 suspected melanomas, were detected in 2,239 persons examined; 30 had probable skin cancer. In another study of 2,000 persons, 16 had malignant melanoma.

Many who attended the various clinics had been aware of a growth for months. They were finally motivated to seek medical attention by advance information disseminated by posters, newsletters, pamphlets, and the various media detailing signs and risks of skin cancer. The convenience of location and the minor cost, if any, prompted many of these people to attend and then to seek further needed care.

Individuals, physicians, organizations, or agencies who wish to implement such clinics in their areas can contact The Skin Cancer Foundation for guidelines, educational materials, and other information. An informed public can stop the spread of skin cancer, a disfigurer and killer. The benefits to all are apparent: savings in total health care, savings in disability and insurance costs, savings in productivity, and best of all, savings in human life.

FURTHERING EDUCATION

Education of children is one of the most neglected areas in cancer prevention programs.

To reduce the incidence of skin cancer and to protect your children's lives and the lives of others, help spread the information you now have to schools, day care centers, nursery schools, and other providers of child care. Enlist their aid in instituting programs geared to a child's understanding.

If you find that your library has few publications, The Skin Cancer Foundation will be glad to provide you with a list of publications and materials, including the brochure "For Every Child Under the Sun." Send a stamped, self-addressed business-size envelope to: The Skin Cancer Foundation, P.O. Box 561, Dept. K, New York, NY 10156. Above all, remember that if you start protecting your child early in life, you can prevent skin cancer later.

CHAPTER

21

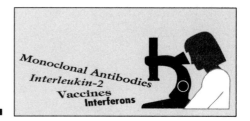

Monoclonal Antibodies
Interleukin-2
Vaccines
Interferons

PROMISING RESEARCH IN MALIGNANT MELANOMA

The only effective treatment for malignant melanoma has been complete surgical excision of early lesions. This has prompted researchers to find a nonsurgical cure, especially for the more advanced lesions. One approach has focused on immunology, the study of resistance to and destruction of organisms and of cellular changes that threaten the body. During the past 40 years, a number of components of the immune system have been identified. This knowledge has led to attempts to harness specific cells and molecules in the fight against disease. The ultimate goal is to develop a way of making the immune system attack specific diseases and disorders, such as melanoma.

Only in the past 5 years has research uncovered real evidence that this goal is attainable. Yet we are only at the tip of the iceberg. The actions of cells and molecules that make up the immune response to disease are so complex, and the reactions to slight changes in this system so profound, that researchers must proceed very carefully.

Until a clearer understanding of the relationship between melanoma and the immune system is developed, surgery, chemotherapy, and radiation therapy will remain the primary weapons against malignant melanoma. In the meantime, we are seeing the development of potential cures that combine traditional treatment with these newer therapies. It must be stressed that all of the potential cures presented in this chapter are in their earliest phases of research, but the promise offered by immunology as a weapon against cancer is very real.

BACKGROUND: THE IMMUNE RESPONSE

The immune system consists of a recognition system combined with an attack and destroy task force.

The recognition system is made up of molecules called antibodies that travel in the bloodstream. Antibodies are large molecules designed to combat specific diseases. The recognition system also includes white blood cells that work together with antibodies to identify intruders that have entered the body, hunting them down and killing them.

Here's an example of how this system works against an invading bacterial or viral infection or a cancer cell.

When a T-cell (helper cell) comes in contact with an invading bacteria or virus, it responds to the foreign molecules—antigens—on the surface of the invader's cell wall (Figure 21.1). The T-cell responds by increasing in number and by stimulating other cells, called B-cells, to produce antibodies.

However, the immune system consists of more than this immediate response to invaders. A series of molecules, called interferons, are also part of the body's response to disease. As

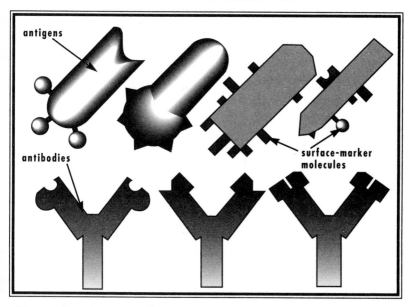

(Figure 21.1) Diagram showing antibodies binding to antigens.

medical researchers gained a greater understanding of the immune system's response to cancer, interferons were the first molecules to be identified as potentially effective in cancer therapy.

INTERFERONS

Interferons are special types of proteins. Their role is to stop viruses from growing, help halt bacterial growth, and adjust the functioning of the immune system. Three types of interferons are produced by different cells in the body.

Interferon alpha is produced by the macrophages, which clean tissues during regular cell maintenance and keep the body free of cellular debris during wound healing, and by blood cells known as lymphocytes. **Interferon beta** is produced by the cells that manufacture collagen. Interferon alpha and beta are very similar in chemical structure, and are called type I interferons. **Interferon gamma**, or type II interferon, is different from the others, and is produced by a type of T-cell.

Interferon gamma seems to play an important role in turning on the immune response to disease. It has been shown to inhibit the growth of melanoma in laboratory experiments.

Experiments have been conducted on cancer patients to study the effectiveness of interferon as an anti-tumor agent. However, interferons do have side effects. Whether administered directly through the veins or by injection into the skin, interferons often produce flu-like symptoms such as fever, chills, fatigue, and muscle aches. These symptoms are related to the amount given but improve with continued treatment. There are other toxic effects on the liver, nervous system, and heart, but these pass after a short time.

Of the type I interferons, interferon alpha may be effective against melanoma. In studies, 15%–25% of patients receiving interferon alpha have responded with a reduction in their tumors, lasting from 6 months to greater than 3 years. These long remissions appear encouraging. Interferon beta has not yet shown consistent anti-tumor effect. With type II interferon, interferon gamma, response rates are similar to those of interferon alpha.

The positive response to type I and type II interferons is better when they are given continuously, and when tumor growth is treated at an early stage. These interferons do not produce dramatic remission in advanced malignant melanoma. They may play an important role, however, following surgical removal of tumors by destroying any cancer cells that remain after surgery.

Combinations of interferons with conventional anti-cancer drugs have shown some success. In addition, combinations of type I and type II interferons and interferons combined with anti-melanoma antibodies are now being studied. It is hoped that this research will lead to a better understanding of the role of interferons in the treatment of malignant melanoma.

VACCINES

The use of vaccines to increase the body's resistance to viral and bacterial infections is well known. This idea is being applied to the development of antibodies and immune cells to fight melanoma through immunization with vaccines containing tumor antigen molecules. It is hoped that the vaccine will stimulate the body to produce antibodies to the tumor and thus start an immune response to tumor cells in much the same way the immune system responds to an invading organism such as a bacterium or a virus.

Vaccines may also help boost cellular immunity, which is thought to play a leading role in resistance to cancer. If effective, vaccines may be used to prevent melanoma, and prevention may be easier to achieve than treatment of established melanoma.

The most convincing evidence that melanoma vaccines are effective comes from animal studies. In one experiment, mice immunized with vaccines made of whole melanoma cells, or melanoma antigens, survived when given lethal doses of melanoma cells that killed non-immunized mice in 6 weeks.

Several medical groups around the country are attempting to develop vaccines to treat human melanoma. So far, the vaccines appear to be safe. Positive results have been reported, particularly in patients with early disease who have previously undergone surgery to remove all evident signs of the melanoma. In some cases, the vaccines seemed to boost immune reactions against melanoma. However, it is still not known if the current generation of vaccines will improve the long-term outlook of melanoma patients.

The technology needed to improve the effectiveness of melanoma vaccines now exists. Intense efforts should, in time, lead to vaccines that can prevent this dreaded cancer.

MONOCLONAL ANTIBODIES

The purpose of a vaccine is to coax the body's B-cells to produce antibodies that will bind to antigen molecules on the cell walls of a particular bacteria or virus, or molecules on the cell wall of a cancer cell. However, it might be possible to bypass the antibody construction process—which can take weeks or months—and directly provide the body with specific antibodies that would work against cancer.

To use the immune system for combating cancer, antibodies must be developed that will attack and help destroy tumor cells but that will not harm normal tissues. An antibody that will bind only one type of antigen molecule is called a monoclonal antibody. To fight cancer, monoclonal antibodies are designed to bind only one type of antigen on the surface of a cancer cell. But to be effective in fighting cancer, there must be enough of these binding sites to trigger an immune system response to the cancer cell. Also, to ensure the safety of normal tissues, the binding site must be unrelated to normal tissues.

Monoclonal antibodies can also be used in other ways to treat melanoma. They can be linked to molecules of other anti-cancer drugs as a way to deliver the drug to tumor sites. Antibodies can also be linked to radio-emitters and used to kill tumor cells more selectively than with conventional radiation therapy. This method could also aid in visualizing the location of tumor nodules in the body.

Monoclonal antibodies can recognize fine differences between antigens, and may prove useful in differentiating between normal and malignant cells for diagnostic studies. Antibodies labeled with radioactive isotopes may help in locating small collections of tumor and improve monitoring of the spread of the disease. Monoclonal antibodies combined with staining systems may help distinguish malignant cells from those that are normal in microscopic examination of biopsy specimens.

INTERLEUKIN-2

Part of the immune system consists of a highly efficient communication system made up of large protein molecules called lymphokines that are produced by helper T-cells. These lymphokines are responsible for activating many cells that participate in the immune response.

In recent animal studies, lymphokine-activated killer (LAK) cells were stimulated with large doses of interleukin-2 (IL-2), a type of lymphokine. When injected into animals, these cells destroyed metastatic tumors.

These results led to the search for a treatment of human tumors using IL-2 and LAK cells. It was discovered that LAK cells could be produced by stimulating lymphocytes from the bloodstream of a normal person. These cells could then be stimulated to kill tumor cells in tissue culture, indicating a potential use of IL-2 and LAK cells in people with cancer. The advent of recombinant DNA technology made the use of IL-2 more feasible by allowing for the production of large quantities of the drug.

Interleukin-2, with or without LAK cells, does have an anti-tumor effect. However, it is potentially quite toxic in high dosages. In several current studies in patients, investigators are evaluating the effectiveness of lower doses given over longer periods of time in the hope of reducing toxic effects.

There are many unresolved issues with this therapy. One is the toxicity of IL-2 that necessitates intensive care monitoring of patients. Another is that the best doses have yet to be identified. Lastly, the therapy must be made less complicated. Nonetheless, the use of IL-2 is promising because of its anti-tumor effect, and malignant melanoma may be one of the cancers that responds best to this therapy.

SUMMARY

Interferons, vaccines, monoclonal antibodies, and interleukin-2 have all shown promise as effective therapies against malignant melanoma. However, these drugs can have very toxic effects, and are only available in a research setting. As with basal and squamous cell carcinoma, prevention and early detection remain the first line of defense against malignant melanoma.

CHAPTER
22

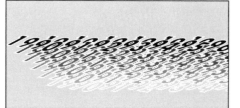

CONCLUSION

The goal of this book has been to provide practical information on the harmful effects of the sun on your skin, with special emphasis on means of prevention, early detection, and treatment of skin cancers.

In the coming years we will undoubtedly see significant advances in skin cancer treatment. We can also look forward to new and improved methods of prevention, including sun protection in the form of a pill!

Although we believe we have covered the topic of skin cancer, in all its aspects, thoroughly, we urge you to discuss any specific issues with your physician. In addition, The Skin Cancer Foundation (Box 561, New York, NY 10156) is an invaluable source of information on the prevention, detection, and treatment of skin cancer: many brochures, posters, newsletters, guidelines, and audiovisual materials are available. You can also contact the American Cancer Society (consult your local phone directory) for materials on skin cancer and the American Academy of Dermatology

(1567 Maple Avenue, P.O. Box 3116, Evanston, IL 60204-3116) for further information about skin conditions and names of dermatologists in your area.

Remember, most skin cancers are preventable. Knowledge and good sun protection habits are your best weapons against the development of skin cancer.

Questions and Answers

1. Can skin cancer recur?

If all the cancer cells have not been removed or destroyed, a cancer may recur. Skin cancers recur more often in areas where they are difficult to remove: the scalp, nose, and ear. Recurrences usually happen within 2 years. For this reason, regular physician follow-up is necessary for 5 years, particularly for persons at high risk. Most sun damage is irreversible; therefore, chances are greater that a new skin cancer will develop in areas of the skin injured by the sun. In 10% of newly diagnosed cases of skin cancer, more than one growth is found.

2. Do you mean that skin cancer can't be cured?

On the contrary, almost all skin cancer that is diagnosed early and treated promptly and appropriately can be cured. This can usually be accomplished without extensive surgery, and with minimal pain and scarring.

3. Will I have a scar?

Any time the skin is cut there will be a scar after healing. The physician will strive to make the scar as unnoticeable as possible.

4. Will surgery disfigure me?

Unless the growth is large and requires extensive repair, there should be no deformity. If the cancer is large, then reconstructive surgery may be necessary, and it will be more difficult to achieve a satisfactory result. In most cases, simple sutures are sufficient to close the wound. In larger wounds, skin flaps or grafts may be necessary. In rare cases of extensive tissue destruction, a prosthesis may be required. Modern surgical techniques have enabled us to produce cosmetically acceptable results.

5. Does the surgery cause much pain or bleeding?

Most skin cancer surgery causes little pain and very little bleeding. We recommend acetaminophen for pain, rather than aspirin. Usually no other pain medication is necessary. Bleeding is minimal. Swelling may occur but soon disappears. If sutures are necessary, they usually remain in place for about 7–14 days. Numbness or sensitivity may occur and persist for up to 2 years. Itching can be soothed with lubricants.

6. Will I need to see my physician after the wound has healed?

About 40% of patients will develop a second skin cancer within 5 years, so careful follow-up is necessary. After two follow-up visits with the surgeon, patients usually can return to their own physician for skin examinations at 6-month intervals.

7. Is there a relationship between skin cancer and the birth control pill?

Although some studies have shown an association between

long-term use of birth control pills and malignant melanoma, it has not been proven conclusively. Nevertheless, women who have other risk factors for skin cancer or other malignancies should discuss use of the pill with their physician.

8. How should I use a sunscreen?

Apply the sunscreen liberally to all exposed areas of skin 30 minutes before sun exposure. Reapply it after swimming or perspiring and while in climates with high humidity. Use a sunscreen all year—in snow, at high altitudes, and even on windy or overcast days. Be sure to pay attention to lips, nose, ear rims, shoulders, back of the neck and legs, tops of feet, and scalp (if bald or if hair is extremely thinned).

9. I have allergies. Can a sunscreen cause an allergic reaction?

If you have allergies, consult with your physician before choosing a sunscreen. Other products, cosmetics, or medications can cross-react with sunscreen ingredients and produce allergic reactions and/or extreme sensitivity to light. These include musk, anthihistamines, antibiotics, tranquilizers, antidiabetic medications, and birth control pills.

10. My doctor says I have a precancer—an actinic keratosis. What does this mean?

Chronic sun exposure can cause blemishes or growths, termed actinic keratoses, which can develop into squamous cell carcinoma. They are scaly, hard lesions that are usually white but may be pink, gray, yellow, or light brown. They may drop off and recur in the same spot. Local destructive therapy is usually sufficient; frequently a biopsy is advisable. Your physician will determine what needs to be done.

11. What are age spots?

So-called "age spots" (sometimes called "liver spots" because of their brown color) are a collection of pigment that appears close to the surface of the skin in the form of unsightly blotches and brown flat patches. Although prevalent on mature skin, they are the result of excessive sun damage, and not of age. They most often appear on sun-exposed parts of the body.

12. Can age spots be removed and, if so, how?

Lentigines or "age spots" are very difficult to remove. Dermabrasion or treatment with liquid nitrogen is sometimes used for this purpose, and some success has been reported with Retin-A cream. Most commercial nonprescription preparations do not work to any significant degree.

13. Why are biopsy and surgical removal necessary for only a very small skin cancer?

A lesion that is tiny on the surface may extend much further below the surface, invading deep into the skin and even organs. A biopsy is necessary to differentiate between types of skin cancer to allow proper treatment. Because skin cancer appears to spread from the outer edge, removal of the entire growth as well as a safety margin of surrounding normal skin is necessary to ensure removal of all cancer cells.

14. Is hospitalization necessary?

Usually surgery can be performed in the physician's office under local anesthetic. Mohs micrographic surgery, in which successive skin layers are removed, stained, and examined for cancer cells, requires up to half a day but is still performed in the physician's office. Extensive surgery for large growths may require hospitalization.

15. Who gets skin cancer?

Anyone can get skin cancer, but it is particularly common in two groups: those who have very fair skin and those who are constantly exposed to the sun, such as sailors, fisherman, gardeners, and construction workers (although indoor workers, who experience intermittent and intense exposure to the sun, are more prone to develop malignant melanoma). Skin cancer also appears to have a hereditary component, and exposure to certain chemicals such as arsenic may trigger skin cancer. Although the disease occurs more frequently in older persons, the damage probably occurs much earlier. Today we are treating many more people in their 20's and 30's.

16. Is age or sex a factor?

If all ages are grouped, more men develop skin cancer than women, but in younger age groups almost as many women develop skin cancer. In men, malignant melanoma is more likely to develop on the chest, shoulders, and back; in women, it develops more often on the legs, perhaps due to patterns of dress. Both sexes develop skin cancer most frequently on the nose. In areas of high sun exposure, as many women as men develop skin cancer, particularly between the third and fourth decades of life. Sun-induced damage to the skin is cumulative; skin cancer develops when a damage threshold is reached.

17. How is skin cancer treated?

Treatment for skin cancer is determined by the type, location, and extent of the cancer, age of the patient, and previous history of skin cancer. A biopsy is taken from the lesion to determine whether it is malignant. If so, the skin cancer may be removed by one of several methods: excisional surgery, curettage-electrodesiccation, cryosurgery, radiation therapy, topical chemotherapy, or by Mohs micrographic surgery.

In excisional surgery, the entire growth and a safety margin at its base and edges are removed. The removed tissue is microscopically examined to ensure that all cancerous tissue has been removed. In curettage-electrodesiccation a curette is used to scrape away the growth, and electrodesiccation is used to burn a safety margin. In cryosurgery, liquid nitrogen applied repeatedly in a freeze-and-thaw cycle destroys cancerous tissue, usually within 24 hours. In radiation therapy, x-rays are beamed at the growth. Many doses are required, and treatment may take weeks or months. In chemotherapy, 5-fluorouracil applied as a cream or ointment is very effective in treating precancerous or superficial lesions. Mohs surgery cuts away thin layers of skin until only healthy tissue remains. Most techniques can be done in the doctor's office, and all have high cure rates.

18. Are there different types of skin cancer?

There are three main types of skin cancer: basal cell carcinoma, squamous cell carcinoma, and malignant melanoma. Each tumor is named for the type of skin cell from which it originates.

The most common type is basal cell carcinoma, which represents 80% of all skin cancers reported yearly in the United States. It appears as a persistent, nonhealing sore or as a red, irritated patch that may crust or itch. It may be a smooth growth with a rolled border, sometimes with visible blood vessels; a shiny bump that is either pink, brown, red, white, or pearly; or, a scarlike, waxy area of skin.

Squamous cell carcinoma is usually a fast-growing, shallow, crusted ulcer with a wide raised border. It can metastasize and may be fatal, although this is rare. It is the second most common skin cancer.

Malignant melanoma is often difficult to distinguish from an ordinary harmless mole. It usually does not hurt, itch, or bleed. Characteristically, the growth is asymmetrical and variegated in color, with irregular borders. Malignant melanoma usually enlarges rapidly and metastasizes, first to local lymph nodes and eventually to body organs. Although it is relatively uncommon, its incidence is growing alarmingly; an individual born today in the United States has a 1 in 120 lifetime risk of developing melanoma. This is the most deadly form of skin cancer.

19. Are sunglasses really important?

Absolutely. Our eyes have some natural protection: the pupils contract in bright light to decrease the amount of light that reaches the retina, and the cornea and lens block some visible radiation. Nonetheless, corneal inflammation can develop from sun exposure, and evidence also implicates solar radiation as the cause of cataracts. The area around the eyes is a common site for skin cancer as well.

The best sunglasses allow only 5% of visible light and infrared radiation to penetrate the eyes. The darkest sunglasses are not the best, because pupils open wider to permit vision, thus allowing more radiation to be transmitted to the retina. An optician, optometrist, or ophthalmologist can assist you in selecting a shade of brown, gray, or green high-contrast lenses that look good and protect you as well.

20. Can tanning lotions and pills be used safely?

No. Tanning lotions are used to facilitate and sometimes hasten tanning. Most are oils with coloring agents that do not protect you at all from ultraviolet radiation. Indeed, you may burn severely. Tanning pills contain chemicals, usually beta-carotene or canthaxanthin, that bronze the skin artificially. These chemicals are approved by the FDA as coloring agents in some foods in small amounts that are not considered dangerous. The amounts contained in tanning pills are much greater and may leave deposits in blood, skin, fatty tissue, and organs such as the liver and kidney. The skin may yellow, and crystalline deposits may form in the eyes. Tanning pills can be dangerous, are illegal in the United States, and provide little protection from the sun.

21. How can I tell if my tanning salon is a good one?

The answer is simple. No tanning salon is good. All tanning lamps emit damaging ultraviolet radiation, no matter what the proportions of UVA and UVB. Tanning salons appear and disappear with such rapidity that policing is almost impossible. Sometimes, personnel are untrained or uninformed; thus, their claims are often misleading. You jeopardize your skin, eyes, and general health by patronizing tanning salons.

22. Can children get skin cancer?

Although skin cancer is uncommon in children, skin damage that later results in skin cancer is accumulated in childhood. A child's skin, particularly an infant's skin, is even more sensitive than adult skin to solar radiation. On the average, children are in the sun 3 times as much as adults are; thus it is vital that their skin be protected from an early age.

Evidence indicates that a single intense sunburn in childhood may double the risk of developing malignant melanoma later in life.

23. If I restrict sun exposure, then how will I get vitamin D?

It is true that we need vitamin D to allow our bodies to absorb calcium and phosphorus and thus to develop strong bones and teeth, and that the sun stimulates a precursor (pro-vitamin D) in our skin cells to produce this necessary vitamin. Today, however, most of us obtain all we need from fortified milk and foods. Synthetic vitamin D in liquid, capsule, or tablet form is an acceptable substitute. Moreover, 10–15 minutes of sun exposure daily will supply ample vitamin D for the body's needs, and even this is not necessary for those who have normal diets.

24. How should I treat a sunburn?

Burns can't always be avoided. If you burn, use cool, wet compresses—either tap water or Burow's solution (available in drugstores diluted with water 40 to 1)—for 20 minutes 4 or 5 times daily to reduce redness and swelling. Coat the burned area lightly with hydrocortisone cream 1/2%, aloe vera, or baby lotion to relieve burning, dryness, and itching. Do not use butter or heavy ointments. Take aspirin or acetaminophen for pain as needed. Drink plenty of fluids to replace moisture loss. Avoid sun exposure until your skin heals completely—from several days to one week. Sun-damaged skin is more susceptible to subsequent burns. If the burn is severe, consult a physician.

25. How do I perform a total body skin examination?

A total body skin examination is a visual self-examination of all cutaneous areas, from scalp to toes. You can perform it easily in a well-lit room with a full-length mirror, a hand mirror, and a hair dryer, by examining your skin systematically. The dryer is used to part your hair and the mirrors to inspect hard-to-see areas. You may need the help of a friend or relative. Once you are aware of the normal condition of your skin, you will more easily note new growths or change in existing growths. Do this at least once a year—more frequently if you have had previous skin cancer or a family history of skin cancer. Consult a physician immediately if you note a suspicious lesion. Ask your physician to examine your skin during your regular physical examination.

26. Is skin cancer contagious?

No. Skin cancer can't be "caught" like a cold. You can't get skin cancer by being with someone who has had it or by sharing something the person uses. Heredity evidently plays a role, however. If family members or grandparents have or have had skin cancer, you have an increased likelihood of developing skin cancer at some time and should be more wary of other risk factors, such as sun exposure, that may increase your vulnerability.

27. Does geography play a role in skin cancer?

Yes. The sun gets more intense as you get closer to the equator: the more intense the sun, and the more sunny days there are, the greater the incidence of skin cancer due to sun exposure alone.

28. What does skin cancer look like?

Skin cancer takes many forms and in its early stages may

appear innocuous to the untrained eye. Skin cancers may be one or several colors, translucent, or pearly. They may be flat, elevated, or bumpy. Suspect growths are those that change rapidly in size, texture, shape, or consistency. New growths that appear after the age of 20 are also suspect. Learn the signs of skin cancer and the normal condition of your skin. Examine your skin closely once a year, and more often if you have had a previous skin cancer or other skin disease, or a family history of malignancy.

Glossary

Actinic (solar) keratosis—Pinkish, scaling "rough" spots caused by prolonged sun exposure. They are considered to be precancerous.

Antibody—A part of the body's defense mechanism that is formed in response to a foreign antigen. Antibodies attack infectious and toxic substances.

Antigen—A molecule found on the cell wall of a bacteria or virus that stimulates the body to produce a specific antibody.

Arsenical keratosis—A horny skin growth most frequently found on the palms and the soles of the feet, caused by exposure to arsenic or use of products containing arsenic, such as Fowler's solution and products for Asian flu.

Basal cell carcinoma—A malignancy made up of cells resembling the basal cells found in the lowest level of the skin. It is the most common form of skin cancer.

Basosquamous cell carcinomas—A skin cancer containing cells having the appearance of both basal cell and squamous cell carcinoma.

Biopsy—A sample of tissue removed from a suspicious area that is sent to the laboratory for microscopic examination and diagnosis.

Birthmark—A noncancerous pigmented spot on the body present since birth. Pigmented nevi and hemangiomas are examples. Very large birthmarks may have an increased risk of developing malignant melanoma.

Bowen's disease—An early form of skin cancer in which growth of the tumor is limited to the surface of the skin.

Carcinogen—A chemical or irritant believed to cause cancer. Examples are soot, charcoal, cigarette smoke, asbestos, arsenic.

Carcinoma—A group of abnormal cells that grow out of control of the body's normal regulatory systems. These cells may spread to other parts of the body, destroying healthy tissue.

Cherry hemangioma—A bright red, circumscribed growth composed of small dilated blood vessels.

Collagen—A protein that serves as the building material of connective tissue.

Comedone—A blackhead, frequently found in people who have acne.

Cryosurgery—A method of treating benign or malignant skin lesions by freezing, usually with liquid nitrogen.

Curettage—A method of removing tissue by scraping it with a special instrument that has a small sharp ring at one end.

Cutaneous—Of or pertaining to the skin, from the word cutis, meaning skin.

Cutaneous horns—Horny growths on the skin.

Dermatologist—A physician who has special training in the diagnosis and treatment of skin diseases.

Dermatology—The medical study of health and disease of the skin.

Dermatopathologist—A physician who specializes in and has had special training in microscopic examination of the skin.

Dermatosurgeon—A dermatologist specializing in skin surgery.

Dermis—The layer of the skin directly below the surface layer (epidermis).

Dysplastic nevi—Unusual or atypical moles that may be markers for an increased risk of melanoma.

Eczema—A common superficial inflammation of the skin, frequently seen as a rash.

Elastosis—A breakdown of the elastic fibrous elements of the skin, resulting in sagging and drooping skin. This is usually caused by excessive sun exposure.

Electrodesiccation—One of the most common methods of treating benign and malignant lesions. The lesion is destroyed by burning or drying the skin with an electric needle.

Epidermis—The outside layer of the skin.

Epithelioma—A term referring to epidermal growths that may be either benign or malignant.

Erythema—Redness on the skin usually produced by blood cells rushing to an area that is inflamed, infected, or damaged by the sun.

Erythroplasia de Queyrat—A form of Bowen's disease (superficial skin cancer) found on the glans of the penis or the lip of the vulva.

Etiology—The cause or causes of a disease.

Estrogen—A female hormone produced primarily by the ovaries.

Excision—Cutting out tissue.

5-Fluorouracil—A chemical preparation used on the skin to destroy precancerous cells.

Granulation—New tissue made by the body to fill in wounds.

Hair follicles—A component of the skin that produces hair.

Herpes simplex—A common skin infection caused by a virus (fever blister, cold sores).

Interferons—Special types of proteins produced by the immune system to stop the growth of viruses and bacteria.

Interleukin-2—A large protein molecule produced by T-cells that activates other cells in the immune system.

Keloid—An overgrown scar at a treated site that extends far beyond the original surgical borders. A hypertrophic scar, on the other hand, is a large scar that remains within the surgical borders.

Keratin—A protein that is the principal component of skin, hair, and nails.

Keratoacanthoma—A rapidly growing benign skin tumor difficult to differentiate from squamous cell carcinoma both in appearance and microscopically.

Keratosis—A type of skin lesion in which there is overgrowth of horny tissue on the skin (see actinic or solar keratosis).

Lentigo—A benign flat brown spot occurring on the skin, commonly referred to as an "age spot" or "liver spot." About 80% of elderly people have them, but they may also occur in younger people as a result of excessive exposure to the sun.

Lesion—A term used to describe a condition restricted to a specific area, which differs from the normal state. A lesion is usually caused by disease.

Leukoplakia—White patches on mucous membranes, usually on the lips, lining of the mouth, tongue, or vagina that are often premalignant.

Liquid nitrogen—A liquefied gas that is very cold. It is often used to freeze and destroy benign and malignant skin tumors.

Lymph vessels—Vessels containing a clear liquid that bathes body cells.

Malignant—Cancerous.

Malignant melanoma—The most serious form of skin cancer composed of malignant pigment cells called melanocytes. These tumors often meet the ABCD criteria: Asymmetric, Border irregularity, Color variability (multiple shades of brown, blue, black, red, white), Diameter greater than one-quarter inch.

Melanin—Pigment that gives us our skin, hair, and eye color. The skin makes more melanin when damaged by the sun.

Melanocytes—The cells in the body that make melanin pigment responsible for color of the skin and hair.

Metastasis—Spread of cancer cells from one part of the body to another, usually via the blood or lymph vessels.

Milium—A whitehead.

Mohs micrographic surgery—A surgical method of removing skin cancer using microscopic control of each layer of tissue as it is removed.

Monoclonal antibodies—Molecules that bind to only one type of antigen. Previously used to diagnose diseases, monoclonal antibodies are now being studied as a treatment for malignant melanoma.

Mortality rate—The number of deaths per year per 100,000 population due to a specific cause.

Nevus (pl. nevi)—A pigmented or unpigmented common mole on the skin.

Nodule—A rounded growth that protrudes above the surface of the skin.

Oncologist—A physician who specializes in the diagnosis and treatment of cancers or tumors.

Ozone layer—The atmospheric layers formed by a photochemical reaction between oxygen and solar radiation. The ozone layer absorbs ultraviolet rays and thus helps shield the earth.

PABA—Paraminobenzoic acid, a common ingredient in sunscreens.

Papule—A small bump on the skin. Skin cancers may initially appear as papules.

Photosensitivity—Low tolerance to light.

Polymorphous light reaction—A skin disease in which exposure causes a variety of skin rashes including hives, bumps or patches of different sizes, or just redness.

Psoriasis—A type of chronic, scaly, hereditary skin disease that is not malignant.

Radiation therapy—Use of x-rays to destroy benign and malignant growths.

Radium—A radioactive element sometimes used in the treatment of cancer.

Reconstruction—The repair of defects on the skin after the removal of a lesion(s).

Retin-A—A drug used to treat acne that has also shown some success in eliminating the fine skin wrinkles caused by sun exposure.

Scleroderma—A disease producing chronic hardening and thickening of the connective tissue, affecting the skin and other organs.

Seborrheic keratoses—Benign, warty skin growths, usually occurring in middde-aged and older people. They appear as numerous yellow or brown raised spots of crusty or irregular texture; they have a "stuck on" appearance as if glued to the skin.

Skin tag—A harmless fleshy growth of excess skin that is found primarily on the armpits and sides of the neck.

Solar radiation—Light rays, both visible and invisible, produced by the sun.

Squamous cell carcinoma—A skin cancer made up of cells resembling those found in the mid-portion of the epidermis.

Stratum corneum—The rough or scaly outermost layer of the epidermis.

Subcutis—The layer of fat just under the skin.

Telangiectasia—Abnormal dilated superficial blood vessel or collection of blood vessels appearing as a red tracery on the skin.

Ultraviolet rays—Waves shorter than visible light, either from the sun or from an ultraviolet source, that can damage the skin.

Urticaria—Hives.

UVA—Ultraviolet light made up of rays that have a wavelength just short of visible light, also referred to as "near-UV" or "long-wave UV."

UVB—Ultraviolet light made up of rays that have a wavelength shorter than UVA. Both UVA and UVB can cause sunburn and skin cancer.

Resources

Actinic Keratoses. Arthur K. Balin, M.D., Ph.D., Andrew N. Lin, M.D. and Loretta Pratt, M.D. Journal of Cutaneous Aging & Cosmetic Dermatology 1:77–86, 1988.

Cancer Incidence and Mortality in the United States. U.S. Department of Health and Human Services, NIH publication no. 85-1837, November 1984.

Cancer Statistics Review, 1973-1986. NIH Publication no. 89-2789, May 1989.

Don't Take the Small Fry Lightly. Henry E. Wiley III, M.D. Skin Cancer Foundation Journal VII:7,65, 1989.

Effective Eye Protection. René Rodriguez-Sains, M.D. Skin Cancer Foundation Journal V:27,71, 1987.

Exploring Behavioral Approaches to UV Risk Reduction. Joseph 5. Rossi. In A. Moshell & L.W. Blankenbaker (Eds.), Sunlight, Ultraviolet Radiation, and the Skin (91-93). Bethesda, M.D., National Institutes of Health, 1989.

Guidelines for the Use of Topical Tretinoin (Retin-A) for Photoaged Skin. Albert M. Kligman, M.D., Ph.D. Journal of the American Academy of Dermatology 21:650–654, 1989.

The Human Immune System: The New Frontier in Medicine. Steven Mizel, M.D., and Peter Jaret. New York, Simon and Schuster, 1986.

Incidence of Nonmelanoma Skin Cancer in the United States. U.S. Department of Health and Human Services, NIH publication no. 83-2433, April 1983.

Long Term Recurrence Rates in Previously Untreated (Primary) Basal Cell Carcinoma: Implications for Patient Follow-Up. Dan E. Rowe, M.D., Raymond J. Carroll, Ph.D., and Calvin L. Day, M.D. Journal of Dermatologic Surgery and Oncology 15:3, March 1989.

The Melanoma Letter. Published quarterly by The Skin Cancer Foundation.

Mohs Surgery is the Treatment of Choice for Recurrent (Previously Untreated) Basal Cell Carcinoma. Dan E. Rowe, M.D., Raymond J. Carroll, Ph.D., and Calvin Day, M.D. Journal of Dermatologic Surgery and Oncology 15:4, April 1989.

Painful Sunburns in Childhood and Adolescence: A possible cause of malignant melanoma. Arthur J. Sober, M.D. and Robert Lew, Ph.D. Skin Cancer Foundation Journal 53,54, 1985.

A Pioneering Program in Early Detection. Denise Andriello Higgins. Skin Cancer Foundation Journal V:13, 14, 1987.

The Presun Report: American Attitudes Towards Sun Exposure. For Westwood Pharmaceuticals by Research & Forecasts, Inc. February 1987.

Prevention of Skin Cancer. Vincent A. DeLeo, M.D. Skin Cancer Foundation Journal VI:15,74, 1988.

Principles of Immunology and Immunodiagnostics. Ralph M. Aloisi. Philadelphia, Lea & Febiger, 1988.

The Rate of Malignant Melanoma in the United States: Are we making an impact? Darrell S. Rigel, M.D. Journal of the American Academy of Dermatology 17:1050–1053, 1987.

Risk Reduction for Nonmelanoma Skin Cancer with Childhood Sunscreen Use. Robert S. Stern, M.D., Milton C. Weinstein, Ph.D., and Stuart G. Baker, ScD. Archives of Dermatology 122:537–545, 1986.

Skin Cancer and Artificial Sources of UV Radiation. Warwick L. Morrison, M.D. Skin Cancer Foundation Journal VI:17,81, 1988.

Skin Cancer in Black Americans: a review of 126 cases. Ki Moon Bang, Ph.D., Rebat M. Halder, M.D., Jack E. White, M.D., Calvin C. Sampson, M.D., and Jerome Wilson, Ph.D. Journal of the National Medical Association 79:51–58, 1987.

Sun & Skin News. Published quarterly by The Skin Cancer Foundation.

The Sun and Sunscreen Protection: recommendations for children. Sidney Hurwitz, M.D. Journal of Dermatologic Surgery and Oncology 14:657–660, 1988.

Sunlight, Ultraviolet Radiation, and the Skin. Program, NIH Consensus Development Conference, May 1989.

Sunscreens and Their Use in the Preventive Treatment of Sunlight-Induced Skin Damage. Madhu A. Pathak, M.B., M.S.(Tech), Ph.D. Journal of Dermatologic Surgery and Oncology 13:739–750, 1987.

Tanning Trends: results from a Skin Cancer Foundation survey. Health, 57–62, May 1988.

Total-Body Photographs of Dysplastic Nevi. William Slue, Alfred W. Kopf, M.D., and Jason K. Rivers, M.D., FRCPC. Archives of Dermatology 124:1239–1243, 1988.

Treatment of Photodamaged Facial Skin with Topical Tretinoin. James J. Leyden, M.D., Gary L. Grove, Ph.D., Mary J. Grove, M.Ed., E. George Thorne, M.D., and Laura Lufrano, M.S. Journal of the American Academy of Dermatology 21:638–644, 1989.

Ultraviolet Radiation and Melanoma: With a Special Focus on Assessing the Risks of Stratospheric Ozone Depletion. Janice D. Longstreth, Ph.D., Editor. Washington, D.C., U.S. Environmental Protection Agency, December 1987.

Educational Materials Available from The Skin Cancer Foundation

You may obtain a free copy of any of the brochures listed below by sending a stamped, self-addressed, business-size envelope for each brochure you request to:

The Skin Cancer Foundation
Box 561, Dept. RB
New York, NY 10156

IT'S NEVER TOO EARLY TO STOP SKIN CANCER — OR TOO LATE: Basic information about skin cancer — the early warning signs, treatment, prevention, sun protection, and sunscreens.

TYPES AND DESCRIPTIONS OF SKIN CANCERS: Six color photographs of the three major types of skin cancer and three examples of precancers, with a brief description of each.

THE ABCD'S OF MOLES AND MELANOMAS: A color brochure comparing four distinctive characteristics of benign and malignant skin growths. A handy visual guide to early recognition. Twelve color photographs.

DYSPLASTIC NEVI AND MALIGNANT MELANOMA, A PATIENT'S GUIDE: Twelve-page color brochure, written in non-technical language, which serves as an aid in recognizing and managing dysplastic nevi. Twelve color photographs.

BASAL CELL CARCINOMA, THE MOST COMMON CANCER: Six-page color brochure with ten photographs depicting the warning signs of this form of skin cancer. Explains the main cause, risk factors, and treatment methods.

SQUAMOUS CELL CARCINOMA: Describes the second most common form of cancer — its causes, clinical manifestations, risk factors and methods of treatment. Six color photograhs.

FOR EVERY CHILD UNDER THE SUN: A GUIDE TO SENSIBLE SUN PROTECTION: Eight-page color brochure offering a ten-step family sun protection program and information on common misconceptions about sun and on the use of sunscreens.

SIMPLE GUIDELINES: Offers twelve simple rules for protection against the sun's damaging rays.

The Skin Cancer Foundation also has the following audiovisual presentations available for purchase (contact the Foundation for information on prices):

SKIN CANCER: PREVENTABLE AND CURABLE (15-minute slide presentation): Covers prevention, detection, treatment and causes of skin cancer. Audio cassette and written script are provided.

SKIN CANCER: PREVENTABLE AND CURABLE (video): a 15-minute presentation suitable for all ages, narrated by television talk show host Dick Cavett. Covers the same topics as slide presentation, including information on sun protection and use of sunscreens, instructions for a total body skin exam, and more. (VHS only)

For a catalog describing all public information materials available from The Skin Cancer Foundation, including the annual Journal, Sun & Skin News, The Melanoma Letter, posters, a skin cancer screening manual, audio/visuals, and additional publications, send a separate stamped, self-addressed, business-size envelope to the Foundation c/o the address above.

Index

Conjunctiva, sun damage to, 81
Conlin, Sandy, 172–73
Contraceptive agents, cancer and, 216–17
Cornea, sunlamp damage to, 60
Corneocytes, 16
Cosmetic procedures, 186–89
Cryosurgery, 137–38
Curettage, 135–36
  biopsy by, 92
  Mohs surgery and, 157
Cutaneous, 16

Dandruff, 16
Deformity from surgery, 216
Dentist's x-ray injury and cancer, 164–65
Dermabrasion, 187
Dermatitis, sunscreens and, 72
Dermatologist, 228
Dermatopathologist, 101, 228
Dermatosurgeon, 228
Dermis, 15, 16
  aging of, 185
Disfigurement from surgery, 216
Drugs:
  melanoma and, 117
  photosensitivity and, 42
  tanning, 76, 222

Ear cancer, 125
Eczema, 228
Education on skin cancer, 126, 200
Educational materials, 237–39
Elastosis, 228
  solar, 185
Electrodesiccation, 134–36
Electromagnetic radiation, 24–25
Electron beam therapy, 133–34
Electrosurgery, 134–36
Epidermis, 15–16
  aging of, 185
Epithelialization, 147
Epithelioma, 228
  basal cell. See Basal cell carcinoma.

Erythema, 40, 228
  minimal dose (MED) for, 47–49
  SPF and, 51–52
Erythroplasia de Queyrat, 91, 228
Escalol 507, 70
Estrogen, 228
Etiology, 228
Examination, skin, 193–200
  cancer signs and, 196
  chart for, 194
  community and workplace, 199–200
  equipment for, 197
  frequency of, 193
  melanoma and, 116–17
  normal blemishes and, 195
  personal story on, 169–70
  professional, 199
  technique of, 197–99, 224
Excision, 131–33
  advantages, 132–33
  biopsy by, 92
  disadvantages, 133
  Mohs surgery and, 158
  recommendations, 133
  technique, 131–32
Eye:
  sunlamps and, 60
  sunlight damage to, 81–83
Eyewear:
  standards for, 83–84
  sunlamps and, 58

Facelifts, 187–88
Fatty layer, 15, 16
Fears, Thomas R., 121
Fibroepithelioma, 98
Flaps, 149–50
5-Fluorouracil (5-FU), 138–40
Follow-up care, 152
Fraumeni, Joseph F., Jr., 121
Freckle, melanotic, 113–14
Freezing, therapy by, 137

Gender. See Sex differences in cancer data.

interferons and, 206–7
interleukin-2 and, 210
lentigo maligna, 113–14
monoclonal antibodies and, 209
mucous membrane, 114
nevi (moles) and, 109–10
nodular, 113
personal stories on, 169–71,
  173–74
protecting yourself from,
  115–18
research in, 203–10
risk factors for, 107, 118
sunlight and, 107–9
superficial spreading, 113
surgical excision of, 133
thickness of, 112
vaccines for, 207–8
warning signs, 116, 117
Melasma, 67
Men. *See* Sex differences in
  cancer data.
Mercury lamps, 57
Metastasis, 95
Methoxsalen, 8-methoxypsoralen,
  76
Micrographic surgery. *See* Mohs
  micrographic surgery.
Milium, 229
Mohs, Frederic E., 156
Mohs micrographic surgery,
  130–31, 155–66
  advantages, 155–56, 160
  case histories, 163–66
  disadvantages, 160
  history of, 156–57
  technique, 157–60
Moles. *See* Nevi.
Monoclonal antibodies, 208–9
Moon children, 42
Mortality rate, 229
Mouth, leukoplakia of, 91
Mutations, cancer and, 95–96

Nevi, 109–11
  basal cell, 99

congenital, 110–11
dysplastic, 109–10
personal stories on, 170–71,
Nodules, 230
  cancerous, 97–98
  melanoma, 113

Oncologist, 230
Oxsoralen, 76
Ozone layer, 31–34

PABA, 68–69
Padimate-O, 70
Pain, surgical, 216
Papule, 230
Para-aminobenzoic acid, 68–69
Parlors, tanning, 55–61, 222
  medical viewpoint on, 59–60
  operators' defense of, 55–59
  protective steps for, 61
  regulations for, 60–61
Patch test, 73
Patient stories, 169–76.
Peels, chemical, 186–87
Personal stories, 169–76
Perspiration, 18–19
Photoaging, 185–86
Photodermatitis, 72
Photosensitivity, 42
Pigmentation, 18. *See also*
  Melanoma, malignant; Nevi.
  cancer and, 9, 98
  tanning and, 40, 46
Pills, tanning, 76, 222
Polymorphous light reaction, 230
Porphyria, 76
Potts, Percival, 6
Pratt, Sharon, 173–74
Preauricular area, grafts from, 149
Precancerous growths, 87–92,
  217–18
  diagnosis and biopsy, 92
Proud flesh, 147
Psoralens, 76
Psoriasis, 230